Clinical Nurse Specialist Addendum

Patricia S.A. Sparacino RN, MS, FAAN
Nancy A. Stotts RN, EdD, FAAN

January 2003

Please direct your comments and/or queries to:

IREC@ana.org

The health care services delivery system is a volatile marketplace demanding superior knowledge, clinical skills, and competencies from all registered nurses. Nursing autonomy of practice, and nurse career marketability and mobility in the new century hinge on affirming the profession's formative philosophy which places a priority on lifelong commitment to the principles of education and professional development. The knowledge base of nursing theory and practice is expanding, and while care has been taken to ensure the accuracy and timeliness of the information presented in the *Clinical Specialist Addendum*, clinicians are advised to always verify the most current national treatment guidelines and recommendations, and to practice in accordance with professional standards of care with regard to the unique circumstances that apply in each practice situation. In addition, every effort has been made in this text to insure accuracy and, in particular, to confirm that drug selections and dosages are in accordance with current recommendations and practice, including the ongoing research, changes in government regulations and the developments in product information provided by pharmaceutical manufacturers. However, it is the responsibility of each nurse to verify all information and to practice in accordance with professional standards of care. In addition, the editors wish to note that provision of information in this text does not imply an endorsement of any particular procedures or services.

Therefore, the authors, editors, American Nurses Association (ANA), American Nurses Association's Publishing (ANP), American Nurses Credentialing Center (ANCC) and the Institute for Research, Education and Consultation cannot accept responsibility for errors or omissions, or for any consequences or liability, injury and/or damages to persons or property from application of the information in this manual and make no warranty, express or implied, with respect to the contents of the *Clinical Specialist Addendum*

Published by: Institute for Research, Education and Consultation at
                 The American Nurses Credentialing Center
                 600 Maryland Avenue, SW - Suite 100 West
                 Washington, DC 20024-2571
                 Phone: (202) 651-7000
                 Internet Address: www.nursecredentialing.org

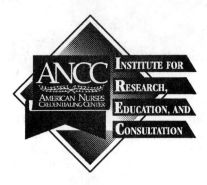

The Institute for Research, Education and Consultation supports the mission of ANCC and benefits consumers and health care providers by

- Inspiring
- Advancing
- Enabling, and
- Demonstrating

The value and power of credentialing.

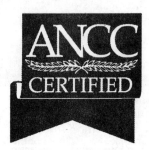

The mission of the American Nurses Credentialing Center is to promote excellence in nursing and health care globally through credentialing programs and related services.

To accomplish its mission, ANCC

- Certifies health care providers,
- Accredits educational providers, approvers, and programs,
- Recognizes excellence in nursing and health care services,
- Educates the public, and collaborates with organizations to advance the understanding of credentialing services, and
- Supports credentialing through research, education, and consultative services.

Clinical Nurse Specialist Addendum

Introduction

This review text has been abstracted, with permission, from *Advanced Nursing Practice: An Integrative Approach (2ⁿᵈ edition)*, edited by Ann B. Hamric, Judith A. Spross, and Charlene M. Hanson, and published by W.B. Saunders. The content has been edited where needed. This condensed version is designed to supply essential content in the support of nurses preparing for certification in specialty nursing as a clinical nurse specialist.

The content addresses advanced practice nurses (APN) in general and clinical nurse specialists (CNS) in particular. Thus the APN label has not been changed. The text has been divided into four parts: Foundations of Clinical Nurse Specialist Practice, Components of Clinical Nurse Specialist Practice, Key APN Competencies as Used by Clinical Nurse Specialists, and The Clinical Nurse Specialist in Action. On page 2, the content table shows the section titles with their original chapter titles and authors.

The CNS role was developed to keep the expert nurse in clinical practice and to improve patient care. The definition of the CNS role has been refined over the years, and the role's evolution has neither been logical nor linear. Yet its effectiveness and survival is derived from its flexibility. We are pleased that you are preparing for this certification examination, the successful completion of which will confirm your competence and establish recognition of your expert practice. Good luck!

Patricia S.A. Sparacino RN, MS, FAAN
Nancy A. Stotts RN, EdD, FAAN

Table of Contents

Foundations of Clinical Nurse Specialist Practice 1

Distinguishing Between Specialization and Advanced Nursing Practice

It is important to distinguish between specialization in nursing and advanced nursing practice. Specialization involves concentration in a selected clinical area within the field of nursing. As the profession has advanced and responded to changes in health care, specialization and the need for the specialty knowledge have increased. Advanced nursing practice includes specialization but goes beyond it. Advanced nursing practice involves expansion, advancement (ANA, 1995; Cronenwett, 1995), and other characteristics in addition to specialization. *Nursing's Social Policy Statement* defined these elements:

> *Expansion refers to the acquisition of new practice knowledge and skills, including the knowledge and skills that legitimize role autonomy within areas of practice that overlap traditional boundaries of medical practice. Advancement involves both specialization and expansion and is characterized by the integration of a broad range of theoretical, research-based, and practical knowledge that occurs as a part of graduate education in nursing* (ANA, 1995, p.14).

APNs are further characterized by their autonomy to practice at the edges of the expanding boundaries of nursing, their predominantly self-initiated treatment regimens, and the greater complexity of their clinical decision making and skill in managing organizations and environments than is seen in basic nursing practice (ANA, 1995).

Defining Advanced Nursing Practice

The concept of advanced nursing practice continues to be defined in various and sometimes contradictory ways in the nursing literature. As the ANA noted, "The term advanced practice is used to refer exclusively to advanced *clinical* practice" (1995, p.15). It therefore seems preferable to define advance nursing without referring to particular roles.

It is also important to advance a definition that clarifies the critical point that advanced nursing practice involves advanced *nursing* skills; it is not a *medical* practice, although APNs perform expanded medical therapeutics in many roles. In addition, advanced nursing practice needs to be defined in a conceptually clear fashion that recognizes the core competencies that all APNs share.

A core definition of advanced nursing practice is proposed, with important assertions as follows:

- Advanced nursing practice is a function of educational and practice preparation *and* a compilation of primary criteria and core competencies.
- Direct clinical practice is the central competency of any APN role.
- All APNs share the same core criteria and competencies, though the actual clinical skill set varies depending upon the needs of the patient population.
- Actual practices differ significantly based on the needs of the specialty patient population served and the organizational framework within which the role is performed.

Conceptual Definition

Davies and Hughes noted, "The term advanced nursing practice extends beyond roles. It is a way of thinking and viewing the world based on clinical knowledge, rather than a composition of roles" (1995, p.157). The ANA's *Scope and Standards of Advanced Practice Registered Nursing* defines the central activities of APNs as follows:

Advanced practice registered nurses manifest a high level of expertise in the assessment, diagnosis, and treatment of the complex responses of individuals, families, or communities to actual or potential health problems, prevention of illness and injury, maintenance of wellness, and provision of comfort. The advanced practice registered nurse has a master's or doctoral education concentrating in a specific area of advanced nursing practice, had supervised practice during graduate education, and has ongoing clinical experiences. Advanced practice registered nurses continue to perform many of the same interventions used in basic nursing practice. The difference in this practice relates to a greater depth and breadth of knowledge, a greater degree of synthesis of data, and complexity of skills and interventions (1996, p.2).

Integrating this understanding with the ANA's components of advanced practice (1995), Hamric conceptualized advanced nursing practice as follows:

Advanced nursing practice is the application of an expanded range of practical, theoretical, and research-based therapeutics to phenomena experienced by patients within a specialized clinical area of the larger discipline of nursing (1996), p.47).[1]

Although graduate education in nursing provides a critical foundation for the expanded knowledge and theory base necessary to support advanced practice, in-depth clinical experiences are equally critical. Indeed, graduate education and clinical practice experience work synergistically to develop the APN. The definition also emphasizes the patient-focused and specialized nature of advanced practice. Finally, the critical importance of ensuring that any type of advanced nursing practice is grounded within the larger discipline of nursing is made explicit.

Advanced nursing practice is further defined by three primary criteria, a central competency, and six core competencies. In reality, these elements are integrated in an APN's practice; they are not separate and distinct features. The essence of advanced nursing practice is found not only in the primary criteria and competencies demonstrated, but also in the synthesis of these elements, along with individual nurse charac-

---

[1] The term "patient" is intended to be used interchangeably with "individual" and "client."

teristics, into a unified composite practice (Davies & Hughes, 1995) that conforms to the conceptual definition.

Primary Criteria

The three primary criteria for advanced practice are an earned graduate degree with a concentration in an advanced nursing practice category, professional certification of practice at an advanced level within a given specialty, and a practice that is focused on patients/clients and their families. These criteria are most often the ones used by states to regulate APN practice, because they are objective and easily measured.

First, the APN must possess an earned graduate (master's or doctoral) degree with a concentration in an APN specialty. Advanced practice students acquire specialized knowledge and skills through study and supervised practice at either the master's or the doctoral level. The content of study includes theories and research findings relevant to the core of the given nursing specialty. The expansion of practice skills is acquired through clinical experience in addition to faculty-supervised practice. As noted previously in the ANA's definition, there is consensus that master's education in nursing is a requirement for advanced nursing practice.

Second, APNs must have professional certification for practice at an advanced level within a specialty. The continuing growth of specialization has dramatically increased the amount of knowledge and experience required to practice safely in modern health care settings. Although the American Nurses Credentialing Center (ANCC) has sponsored CNS certification examinations in medical-surgical and psychiatric areas for years, advanced practice certification examinations in particular specialties such as maternal-child health have been slow to develop. If no certification examination exists for the advanced practice level of a particular specialty, the APN should be certified at the highest level available.

Third, the APN engages in a practice focused on patients and their families. It is critical to promoting clarity about advanced nursing practice that the term be used to describe advanced *clinical* practice (ANA, 1995), and refer to roles that have direct clinical practice as their central focus.

Direct Clinical Practice: The Central Competency

Advanced practice is defined by a set of core competencies that are enacted in each APN role. The term "competency" is used to refer to a defined area of skilled performance. The first core competency of direct clinical practice is central to and informs all of the others. Advanced nursing practice is first and foremost characterized by excellence in direct clinical practice.

Although clinical expertise is a central ingredient of the direct practice competency that defines advanced nursing practice, it is not the sole focus of the clinical practice of APNs. Advanced direct care practice includes five characteristics: (1) use of holistic perspective, (2) formation of partnerships with patients, (3) use of expert clinical reasoning, (4) reliance on research evidence as a guide to practice, and (5) use of diverse health and illness management approaches. Experiential knowledge and graduate education work synergistically to develop these characteristics in an APN's clinical practice.

Core Competencies

Six core competencies further define advanced nursing practice regardless of role function or setting. These competencies have repeatedly been identified as essential components of advanced practice (American Association of Colleges of Nursing, 1995; ANA, 1995; Davies and Hughes, 1995; National Association of Clinical Nurse Specialists, 1998; National Council of State Boards of Nursing, 1993; National Organization of Nurse Practitioner Faculties, 1995; Spross & Baggerly, 1989). They are:

1. Expert guidance and coaching of patients, families, and other care providers
2. Consultation
3. Research skills, including utilization, evaluation, and conduct
4. Clinical and professional leadership, which includes competence as a change agent
5. Collaboration
6. Ethical decision-making skills

Scope of Practice

The term "scope of practice" refers to the legal authority granted to a professional to provide and be reimbursed for health care services. This authority for practice emanates from many sources, such as state and federal laws and regulations, the profession's code of ethics, and professional practice standards. For all health care professionals, scope of practice is most closely tied to state statutes; for nursing, these statutes are the Nurse Practice acts of the various states. An APN's scope of practice is characterized by specialization; expansion of services provided, including diagnosing and prescribing; and autonomy to practice (ANA, 1996). There are differences in the scope of practice among the various APN roles; various specialty organizations have provided detailed and specific descriptions for their specialties. Significant variability in state practice acts continues such that APNs can perform certain activities, notably prescribing medications and practicing without physician supervision, in some states but may be constrained from performing these same activities if they move to another state (Safriet, 1992, 1994). APNs now face new nongovernmental, market-based barriers to their practices.

Operational Definitions of Advanced Nursing Practice

The CNS role has been distinguished by the expectation of practice in four subroles: clinical expert, consultant, educator, and researcher (Hamric & Spross, 1989). The CNS is first and foremost a clinical expert, who provides direct care to patients with complex health problems. CNSs not only learn consultation processes as do other APNs, but also function as formal consultants within their organizations. Their multifocal practice in these different subroles means that CNS practice is fluid and changeable. Developing, supporting, and educating nursing staff; managing system change in complex organizations to build teams and improve nursing practices; and "massaging the system" (Fenton, 1985) to advocate for patients are unique role expectations of the CNS. Expectations regarding research activities have been central to this role since its inception. More recently, the National Association of Clinical Nurse Specialists (NACNS, 1998) has distinguished CNS practice by characterizing "spheres of influence" in which the CNS develops competencies. These include the patient/client sphere, the nursing personnel sphere, and the organization/network sphere.

The blended CNS/Nurse Practitioner (NP) role combines the CNS's in-depth specialized knowledge of a particular patient population with the NP's primary health care expertise. It is important to clarify that CNSs who obtain NP skills are not necessarily functioning in a blended role. Many work as NPs in primary care NP or Acute Care Nurse Practitioner (ACNP) roles as described earlier. The CNS/NP provides primary and specialty care, including clinical management, to a complex patient population, such as children with diabetes. A unique feature of this role is the provision of primary and specialized care such that the blended CNS/NP crosses set boundaries to provide continuity of care. An additional characteristic that distinguishes this role from that of the ACNP is the expectation for CNS competencies in the three spheres of influence noted earlier. For example, this role combines individual patient management with expectations to develop nursing staff as well as to effect change in complex organizational practices. In addition to learning the core advanced practice competencies, education for this role must include functional role preparation for both the CNS and the NP roles. Blended-role APNs also must ensure that their roles are carefully structured to allow time and emphasis in the three spheres of influence.

Concepts that Define Advanced Nursing Practice

The American Nurses Association's (ANA's) *Nursing's Social Policy Statement* identifies and defines three concepts to differentiate advanced nursing practice from basic nursing practice:

- *Specialization* is concentrating or delimiting one's focus to part of the whole field of nursing.
- *Expansion* refers to the acquisition of new practice knowledge and skills, including knowledge and skill legitimizing role autonomy within areas of practice that overlap traditional boundaries of medical practice.
- *Advancement* involves both specialization and expansion and is characterized by the integration of theoretical, research-based, and practical knowledge that occurs as part of graduate education in nursing. (ANA, 1995, p.14)

Practice Models

Benner (1985) described advanced nursing practice expertise in describing the role of the Clinical Nurse Specialist (CNS). She saw CNS expertise as a hybrid of practical knowledge gained from frontline clinical practice and sophisticated skills of knowledge utilization. The CNS has in-depth knowledge of a particular clinical population and grasps in theory and practice the illness and disease trajectory of that patient population.

Fenton (1985) and Brykczynski (1989) each independently applied Benner's model of expertise at the advanced nursing practice level in examining the practice of CNSs and nurse practitioners (NPs), respectively. In a later publication, Fenton and Brykczynski (1993) compared their earlier research findings to identify similarities and differences between CNSs and NPs, using Benner's understanding of the concepts of domains, competencies, roles, and functions.

Others have taken a more deductive approach, first developing a theoretical rationale to explain particular phenomena. In this manner, Calkin (1984) developed a model of nurse administrators to use in determining how to differentiate advanced nursing practice in personnel policies. Calkin illustrated the application of this framework in explaining how APNs perform under different sets of circumstances: when there is a high degree of unpredictability; when there are new conditions or a new patient population or new sets of problems; and when there are a wide variety of health problems, requiring the services of "specialist generalists," as she called them. When a patient's health problems elicit a wide range of human responses with continuing and substantial unpredictable elements, the advanced practice nurse (APN) functions are to:

- Identify and develop interventions for the unusual by providing direct care,
- Transmit this knowledge to nurses and in some settings to students,
- Identify and communicate needs for, or carry out research related to human responses to these health problems,

- Anticipate factors that may lead to the presence of unfamiliar responses,
- Provide anticipatory guidance to nurse administrators when the changes in the diagnosis and treatment of these responses may require altered levels or types of resources (Calkin, 1984, p.28).

The National Association of Clinical Nurse Specialists (NACNS) published a *Statement on Clinical Nurse Specialist Practice and Education* in 1998. In this statement, they moved from an earlier conceptualization of subroles to a complex of:

1. Essential characteristics – a combination of leadership, collaboration, and consultation skills and professional attributes;
2. Spheres of influence – patients/clients, nursing personnel and organizational/network – with outcomes and competencies for each sphere;
3. Content areas for the competencies (NACNS, 1998).

Thus, a virtual matrix was created to serve purposes ranging from making explicit the contributions of CNSs to providing a basis for curricula and certification examinations.

Consensus Building Around Roles and Specialty Scopes

For some time, cross-matching of frameworks has been used to contrast, compare and combine the role of CNS and NP. Now the focus should shift toward bringing the practice of all APNs into conceptual unity. This is not to suggest that the practice is identical for all, but that the common elements should be identified and differences noted.

Attention should be directed to the "scope" dimension of advanced nursing practice. Among its other characteristics, advanced nursing practice is specialized. Most of nursing's specialties have statements of scope, often with associated competencies or functions. The respective scopes of practice in various specialties within advanced practice roles must be addressed and a rationale articulated for further development and refinement.

The ANA's *Scope and Standards of Advanced Practice Registered Nursing* (1996) is a helpful document in striving for consensus among advanced practice roles and specialties. Within that framework, the generic scope and standards deal with the broader field of advanced practice nursing, as the title of the document makes clear, and standards of care have been differentiated from standards of professional performance. Although the professional performance standards focus upon the individual practitioner, they do refer to the individual as a member of the collective profession and open the door to consideration of all that is implied in the professional role relative to foundational factors.

Role Development

In the current managed care environment, the pressure to be cost effective and to make an impact on outcomes is greater than ever. Yet literature indicates that the initial year of practice is one of transition (Brykczynski, 1996) and maximum potential is not reached until approximately five or more years in practice (Cooper & Sparacino, 1990). Professional role development is a dynamic, ongoing process that, once begun, spans a lifetime. Like socialization for other professional roles, the process of becoming an APN involves aspects of adult socialization as well as occupational socialization.

Novice-to-Expert Skill Acquisition Model

Acquisition of knowledge and skill occurs in a progressive movement through stages of performance from novice to expert as depicted by Dreyfus and Dreyfus (1977, 1986). A major implication of the novice-to-expert model for advanced practice nursing is the claim that even experts can be expected to perform at lower skill levels when they enter new situations or positions. Role development is pictured as multiple, dynamic, and situational processes with each new undertaking being characterized by passage through earlier transitional phases with some movement back and forth, horizontally and laterally, as different career options are pursued. Another significant implication of the Dreyfus model for APNs is the observation that performance level also decreases when performers are subjected to intense scrutiny, whether it is their own or someone else's (Roberts, Tabloski, & Bova, 1997). A third implication of this skill acquisition model for APNs is the need to accrue experience in actual situations over time, so that both practical and theoretical knowledge are refined, clarified, personalized, and embodied, forming an individualized repertoire of past experience that guides advanced practice performance.

According to this model, there is a generic process of skill acquisition through which humans proceed in stages from novice to expert as they acquire new psychomotor, perceptual, and judgment skills. The progression from novice level to advanced-beginner level and then to competent level is incremental. There is a change from "acting like", sometimes referred to as the imposter phenomenon (Arena & Page, 1992; Brown & Olshansky, 1997, 1998), to individualized embodiment of the new role as the individual moves up to the proficient level.

The proficient level represents a discontinuous, qualitative leap from the competent level whereby intuition, defined as "holistic situation recognition" (Dreyfus & Dreyfus, 1986, p. 28) replaces analytically reasoned responses. The deep situational understanding associated with expertise involves holistic pattern recognition, described as "the intuitive ability to use patterns without decomposing them into component features" (Dreyfus & Dreyfus, 1986, p.28). Decomposition of situations into abstract attributes is associated with earlier skill levels. The extent of an individual's involvement in a particular situation influences her or his decision-making ability (Benner et al., 1996). Deliberative rationality, or a fine tuning of intuitions, takes place at the expert level, replacing the calculative rationality characteristic of other levels. Deliberative rationality is involved in distinguishing a novel situation or a situation where there is an incorrect initial grasp from a situation in which experience can be trusted.

Role Development Issues

Role ambiguity develops when there is a lack of clarity about expectations, a blurring of responsibilities, uncertainty regarding implementation of subroles, and the inherent uncertainty of the existent knowledge base of a discipline. According to Hardy and Hardy (1988), role ambiguity characterizes all professional positions. They pointed out that role ambiguity may be positive in that it offers opportunities for creative possibilities. Role ambiguity has been widely discussed in relation to the CNS role (Chase et al., 1996; Payne & Baumgartner, 1996; Redekopp, 1997).

Role incongruity is intrarole conflict, which Hardy and Hardy described as developing from two sources. Incompatibility between skills and abilities and role obligations in one source of role incongruity. Another source of role incongruity is incompatibility between personal values, self concept, and expected role behaviors.

Role conflict develops when role expectations are perceived to be contradictory or mutually exclusive. APNs may experience intrarole conflict as well as both inter-and intraprofessional role conflicts. Conflicts between physicians and APNs constitute the most common situations of interprofessional conflict of interest. Major sources of conflict for physicians and APNs are the perceived economic threat of competition, limited resources in clinical training sites, and lack of experience working together.

APNs experience intraprofessional role conflict with other nurses and within the nursing profession for a variety of reasons. Hamric and Taylor (1989) pointed out that staff resistance to change, complacency or apathy, and the fact that nurses are generally not accustomed to seeking consultation from other nurses as experts can impede CNS role development.

Role Transitions

Role transitions are defined here as dynamic processes of change that occur over time as new roles are acquired. Five essential factors found to influence role transitions were noted by Schumacher and Meleis (1994):

1. The personal meaning of the transition, which related to the degree of identity crisis experienced;
2. The degree of planning, which involves the time and energy devoted to anticipating the change;
3. Environmental barriers and supports, which refer to family, peer, school, and other components;
4. Levels of knowledge and skill, which related to prior experience and school experiences;
5. Expectations, which are related to role models, literature, media, and the like.

Role strain or role insufficiency accompanying the transition to APN roles can be minimized, although certainly not completely prevented, by (1) individualized assessment of these five essential factors, (2) development of strategies to cope with them, and (3) rehearsal of situations designed to apply those strategies.

APN graduates can be expected to experience attitudinal, behavioral, and value conflicts as they move from the academic world, where holistic care is highly valued, to the work world, where organizational efficiency is paramount. The process of APN role implementation is an example of a situational transition (Schumacher & Meleis, 1994).

Anticipatory socialization experiences in school can facilitate role acquisition, but they cannot prevent the conflicts that occur with the movement into a new position and actual role implementation. APN role development has been described as dynamic, complex, and situational. It is influenced by many factors, such as experience, level of expertise, personal and professional values, setting, specialty, relationships with co-workers, aspects of role transition, and life transitions.

Components of
Clinical Nurse
Specialist Practice 2

Expert Clinician

Direct Care Activities

Direct care and direct clinical practice refer to the activities and functions APNs enact within the patient-nurse interface.[2] The activities that occur in this interface are unique because they are interpersonally and physically co-enacted with a particular patient for the purpose of promoting the patient's health or well-being. Although other APN activities occurring prior to and adjacent to the nurse-patient interface have a great influence on the direct care that occurs in the interface, they either are not co-enacted with an individual patient or their main purpose is something other than promoting the well-being of the individual patient. In this situation, the APN is engaged in clinical practice but she or he is not providing direct care. Restricting the use of the term "direct care" to what occurs in the patient-nurse interface serves both heuristic and practical purposes.

Among domains of APN practice (Fenton & Brykczynski, 1993), terms that describe the direct care activities of APNs include: diagnostic/patient monitoring, administering/monitoring therapeutic interventions and regimens, helping patients and families during crisis, teaching/coaching, and effective management of rapidly changing situations. Activities and functions such as monitoring/ensuring the quality of health care practices, organization and work role competencies, and the consulting role are recognized as domains of advanced nursing practice contiguous with direct care activities but do not define direct care.

Formation of Partnerships with Patients

Many conceptual models (e.g., Watson's Human Caring theory and the Modeling and Role-Modeling Theory of Erickson, Tomlin, and Swain) propose that forming partnerships with patients will result in improved health outcomes (Erickson, Tomlin, & Swain, 1983; Raudonis & Acton, 1997; Watson, 1997). Based on current knowledge, providers should be reluctant to make any assumptions about an individual patient's preference for participation in clinical decisions regarding how to prevent and diagnose disease, or manage an illness. Instead, they should individually determine each patient's preference for participation in decision-making, and be sensitive to the fact that patients' preferences may change over time as they get to know the provider better and as different kinds of health problems arise. Once the patient's preference has been elicited, the provider should tailor his or her decision-making style to the patient's preference.

---

[2] It is assumed in this definition that "the patient" may be an individual, a family, a community or community group, a workplace or school group, or a health interest group.

Another important factor affecting whether and how persons want to participate in health care decision making is their cultural background. Some groups have ways of thinking and communicating expectations that are quite different from those of the health care provider, and possibly unfamiliar to her or him (Cooper-Patrick et al., 1999; Waite, Harker, & Messerman, 1994). These differences can cause confusion, misunderstandings, and even conflicts that disrupt the patient-provider relationship and discourse. Moreover, they often complicate attempts to resolve misunderstandings because different cultural groups approach conflict negotiation differently.

Some patients are not able to enter fully into partnership with APNs because they are too young, have compromised cognitive capacity, or are unconscious. Although these patients may be limited in their abilities to speak for themselves, they are not entirely without voice. Experts who work with patients who cannot verbalize their concerns and preferences learn to pay close attention to how patients are responding to what happens to them; facial expressions, body movement, and physiological parameters are used to ascertain what causes the patient discomfort and what helps alleviate it (Benner, Tanner, & Chesla, 1996).

Expert Clinical Thinking and Skill Performance

The research on how clinical experts think is less than cohesive. There are two main schools of thought about clinical reasoning, the information-processing school and the intuitive school; both are represented in the current research literature. The information-processing viewpoint is based on the assessment-diagnosis-treatment model of clinical practice and on an information-processing view of clinical judgment (Bulechek & McCloskey, 1999a; Gordon et al., 1994; Narayan & Corcoran-Perry, 1997). Typically, researchers are interested in the cognitive processes practitioners use in bringing clinical knowledge to bear on a particular situation. Researchers in the intuitive, or thinking-in-action, tradition use naturalistic, descriptive, and interpretive methods to study clinical judgment. Those who view clinical judgment through the intuitive lens focus on how the nurse comes to have a deep understanding of a particular patient's evolving situation or unfolding account.

These two views of clinical thinking do not share much common language, and articulation between their research findings is limited. Even though the two views of clinical reasoning are based on different epistemological assumptions, they are not inherently incompatible. It is possible that they focus on different aspects of clinical reasoning, judgment and decision making. For a nurse to acquire a deep and accurate understanding of a situation, these two ways of thinking may need to occur simultaneously and interactively. The intuitive view of clinical thinking may be most useful in portraying how clinicians perceive, make sense of what is occurring, and come to deeply understand a situation in which they are embedded. The information-processing view may enlighten our understanding of the way clinicians activate theoretical, domain-specific knowledge to help make sense of a particular situation.

Clinical Reasoning and Judgment

Specialized knowledge and accrued experience in working with a population of patients lay the foundation for the expert clinical thinking that is associated with advanced direct care practice. Once an APN has been in practice for a while, formalized knowledge and experiential knowledge become so mixed together that they are no longer distinguishable. Importantly, the expert's clinical knowledge is characterized by the ability to make fine distinctions among common features of a particular condition that were not possible during beginning practice. Eventually, the expert's clinical knowledge consists of a complex network of memorable cases, prototypic images, domain-relevant concepts, thinking strategies, moral values, maxims, probabilities, behavioral responses, associations, illness trajectories and timetables, research findings, and therapeutic information. Thus, experts have extensive, varied, and complex knowledge networks that can be activated to help understand clinical situations and events.

Expertise involves more than accumulated stores of knowledge. Clinical reasoning brings together the clinical knowledge of the provider with specific observations, perceptions, events, and facts from the situation at hand to produce an understanding of what is occurring (O'Neill, 1995). Experts have the ability to rapidly scan a situation (e.g., past records, patient's appearance, and the patient's unexpressed concern or discomfort) and identify salient and relevant information. Relying heavily on their perceptions, observations, and physical assessment skills, experts quickly activate one or several lines of reasoning regarding what might be going on. Next, they conduct a more focused assessment to determine which one best explains the situation at hand. These lines of reasoning are really informal, personal theories about the specific patient situation; their formulation draws from personal knowledge of the particular patient, from personal knowledge acquired from past experiences, and from formalized domain-specific knowledge (Narayan & Corcoran-Perry, 1997; Rolfe, 1997a). Most patient accounts unfold in a fairly predictable way, and the APN arrives at a diagnosis and/or intervention with considerable confidence. When there is ambiguity, experts often break into conscious problem solving.

Importantly, knowing the patient may be critical to the nursing functions of surveillance and rescuing. The extent to which a nurse knows the patient may be associated with that nurse's ability to:

- Recognize that risk factors are present
- Detect early indicators of a problem (i.e., a slight change in pattern)
- Take time preventive action

While looking for patterns, the expert nurse is alert to nonfitting data, that is, data that seem important but just do not fit into any of the clinician's explanations of the situation.

The clinical acumen of APNs and the inferences/hypotheses/lines of reasoning they generate are highly dependable. However, as practice becomes repetitive, APNs may develop routine responses that put them at risk of making certain types of thinking errors (Schön, 1984). Errors of expectancy occur when the correct diagnosis is not generated as a hypothesis because there is a set of circumstances, in either the clinician's experience or the patient's circumstances, that predisposes the clinician to disregard it. Erroneous conclusions are also more likely when the situation is ambiguous, that is, when the meaning or reliability of the data is unclear, the interpretation of the data is not clear-cut, the best approach to treatment is debatable, or one cannot say for sure whether the patient is responding well to treatment (Brykczynski, 1991). Poor judgment also can result from tunnel vision; overgeneralization; influence by a recent, dramatic experience; and fixation on certain problems to the exclusion of others (Benner et al., 1999). Faulty thinking is not the only source of error in clinical decision making. Other sources include inaccurate observations, misinterpretation of the meaning of data, a sketchy knowledge of the particular situation, and a faulty model of the disease/condition/response.

Treatment Decisions

The decision whether to treat or not can be complex, because the CNS is faced with a string of probabilities that do not all point to the same decision. The most clear-cut situation is when the condition is assuredly present, a particular treatment is known to be highly effective, the treatment can be expected to be low in risk for the particular patient, and the clinician is comfortable with the treatment. Unfortunately, many (probably most) therapeutic decisions are not so clear-cut. One goal of treatment decision making is to choose from among several possible interventions the one that will have the highest probability of achieving the outcomes the patient most desires. However, another goal is to "particularize" the treatment or action to the individual patient (Benner et al., 1996). Particularizing requires that the final decision factor in:

- The acceptability of the treatment to the patient
- What has worked for the patient in the past
- The patient's motivation and ability to use or follow the treatment
- The likelihood that the patient will continue to use the treatment even if side effects are experienced
- The financial burden of the treatment

Other investigative work has also delineated what is meant by individualized care. Tailoring of care involves components of "knowing the patient": (1) the nurse's understanding of the patient, and (2) the selection of individualized interventions. Knowing the patient may result in expert clinical decision making and positive patient outcomes (Radwin, 1996).

Ethical Reasoning

Clinical decision making is linked inextricably to ethical reasoning. The literature regarding how to resolve ethical dilemma issues is extensive, but "preventive ethics" offers an approach to incorporating ethical considerations into clinical thinking and decision making that makes a great deal of sense. (Forrow, Arnold, & Parker, 1993). This approach places an emphasis on preventing ethical conflicts from developing rather than waiting until a conflict arises; it does so by shaping the process of clinical care so that possible value conflicts are anticipated and discussed prior to outright conflict. In addition to emphasizing early communication between the patient and the provider(s) about values, preventive ethics requires explicit, critical reflection on the institutional factors that lead to conflict (Forrow et al., 1993). Another aspect of preventive ethics is an effort to create and preserve trust and understanding among providers as well as between patients (and their families) and providers. Thus preventive ethics is proactive in that it requires providers to consider how the routine processes of care either foster or prevent conflicts from occurring or at least being identified at an early stage.

Information Management

A final aspect of APN clinical decision making is the increasingly important competency of managing the extensive data and knowledge that are required to base practice on available, current information (Kibbe, 1999).

Use of Research Evidence

Clinical nurse specialists (CNSs) have led efforts in many agencies to move toward research-based practice (Hanson & Ashley, 1994; Hickey, 1990; Mackay, 1998; Stetler, Bautista, Vernale-Hannon, & Foster, 1995).

The Research-Based Practice Process

Bringing research to bear on clinical practice requires systematic, precise analysis and careful consideration of whether and how credible findings should be incorporated into practice. Knowledge of one's clinical practice area and familiarity with its literature are essential to formulating a clinical question for which a body of research evidence can be found. Perhaps the most difficult step for most clinicians is appraising the research evidence, that is, deciding whether a study was well conducted and whether the results are clinically significant (Brown, 1999). Findings are judged to be credible if they were produced by a scientifically sound study and clinically significant if incorporating them into practice is likely to make a difference in patient outcomes. For findings that pass these two screens, it is still necessary to think about what patients in one's own practice would benefit from the research-based change in practice being considered and whether the protocol or intervention would be feasible in the practice setting. A quality improvement project could be planned to evaluate whether the outcomes produced under research conditions have been realized in everyday practice. This evaluation should involve data collection and measurement, but it need not be a research study (Nelson et al., 1998). Measuring results can lead to a better understanding of the extent to which general research knowledge works at the local level. By fine-tuning general knowledge to local conditions, improvement in care and patient outcomes can be realized and documented.

Forms of Research Evidence

The findings of one study, even a well-conducted one, are a limited basis on which to design or change practice. The better strategy is to review all the studies that have examined the clinical issue to determine what common findings have appeared in several settings and with different populations. To keep a research-based practice project feasible, the number of studies included in the review should be limited by an objective method. The best way to limit the number of studies is to focus the clinical question of interest by being specific about what form of intervention or what outcomes you are interested in.

Summaries of many or all studies on clinically relevant topics are appearing in clinical journals with greater frequency. These summaries come in the forms of integrative research reviews, meta-analyses, and research-based clinical guidelines. These summaries, when thoroughly and systematically produced, provide a basis for assessing the scientific knowledge about a particular topic that is superior to only using the findings of one or a few studies. Clinical guidelines also are being produced with increased frequency by clinical specialty organizations as well as government agencies and evidence-based centers. The good ones communicate to the potential user the strength of the evidence for each recommendation (i.e., number and types of studies, expert consensus, logical reasoning).

Theory-Based Practice

Theory often brings together research findings and concepts generated through practice in a way that helps practice be more purposeful, systematic, and comprehensive. The use of conceptual models or theories (e.g., the models of Orem, Newman, and Roy) provide nurses with a broad perspective within which they can view client situations. Conceptual models also help nurses plan and implement care in a purposeful, proactive, and comprehensive manner (Raudonis & Acton, 1997). Their value is enhanced if there is a natural fit between the model and the nature of the clinical issues of the patient population. Theory-based practice is, however, more than the use of conceptual models as a guide to practice. More specific theories, called middle-range theories, guide practice in a different way. Middle-range theories address the experiences of particular patient populations or of a cohort of people who are dealing with a particular health or illness issue (e.g., changing a health-related behavior or coping with postpartum depression). Because middle range theories are more specific in what they explain, CNSs often find them more directly applicable than the conceptual models.

Knowledge-Based Practice

Beyond research-based practice and theory-based practice is the more essential issue of knowledge-based practice. Knowledge is the goal of both the conduct of research and the development of theory. Moreover, acquisition of useful and dependable knowledge requires both research work and theory work. Research findings are bits of knowledge, whereas theories are explanatory systems describing how some aspect of how the world works. The goal is to acquire meaningful and useful knowledge that has been tested using scientific methods and found to be an accurate and useful portrayal of certain realities. APNs have the educational background to appreciate how these two knowledge production pathways of science work together and separately to produce useful and dependable clinical knowledge.

Therapeutic Interventions

There is evidence that APNs use a broad range of interventions, with substantial reliance on self-care and low-technology interventions. APNs' direct care often involves management and/or coordination of complex situations. APNs have been designated the providers responsible for coordinating discharge for patients with complex follow-up care or for conducting patient education with high-risk patients (Damato et al., 1993; Naylor et al., 1999). APNs are assuming management responsibilities for discrete and complex aspects of care, such as care of elderly patients who become confused during hospitalization, pain management in patients who are chronically or terminally ill, skin care for patients at risk for skin break down or delayed healing, and aggressive management of complex cases (Urban, 1997).

Many CNSs have had the experience of being called for a consultation and finding that there is a need for skilled communication, advocacy, or coordination of the various providers' plans – or some combination thereof. The patient may not be progressing because wound care, pain management, and physical therapy have not been well thought out and coordinated. A family may be angry because plans keep changing and they are receiving conflicting information from various providers. Typically, the CNS talks with the patient and family to become familiar with their concerns and objectives, and then brokers a new plan of care that reflects the patient's and family's needs and preferences as well as the clinical objectives of the involved providers (Steele & Fenton, 1988). The agreed-upon plan must also be consistent with the care authorized by the third-party payers for the patient, or a special agreement must be negotiated. This brokering requires broad clinical knowledge regarding the objectives of various providers, interpersonal skill in calming the results of misunderstandings, diplomacy to get the stakeholders to see other points of view, and a commitment to keeping the patient's needs at the center of what is being done.

Clinical nurse specialist care should continue to incorporate the holistic perspective, partnerships with patients, expert clinical reasoning and skilled performance, the use of research-based evidence, and the use of diverse management approaches. Together, these qualities form a solid foundation for providing scientifically based, person-centered, and population-validated health care.

Educator

Numerous factors in contemporary health care have increased the focus on patient education as a means of improving effectiveness and efficiency and achieving cost and quality outcomes. Expert guidance and coaching are key foci of the APN's direct care role. APN's coaching of clients assumes an understanding of basic principles of education and an awareness of the research on which patient education is based. APNs are responsible for knowing the theoretical and scientific bases of patient teaching in their specialties and practice settings.

Coaching is complex interpersonal work that helps people who are facing equally complex personal transitions or journeys. Coaching has been used by several disciplines to describe interactions between experts and learners that focus on developing the learner's knowledge and skill in an area that is within the coach's expertise (Spross, 1994). In cognitive psychology, social skills tutoring (Frisch et al., 1982) and interpersonal cognitive problem solving (Hops, 1983) are coaching techniques that have been used to improve individuals' social skills, language skills, and problem-solving abilities. Both techniques include direct verbal instructions in problem-solving principles. Interpersonal cognitive problem solving also emphasizes thinking processes such as identifying problems, generating alternative solutions, and anticipating the consequences of solutions (Pelligrini & Urbain, 1985). APNs use their knowledge of a patient as well as knowledge from past experiences with similar patients to craft patient-specific coaching interventions.

Transitions

Chick and Meleis offered a clinically useful definition of transitions:

> *Transition is a passage from one life phase, condition, or status to another . . . Transition refers to both the process and outcome of complex person-environment interactions. It may involve more than one person and is embedded in the context and the situation* (1986, pp. 239-240).

Chick and Meleis further characterized the process of transition as having phases during which individuals experience: (1) a disconnectedness from their usual social supports, (2) a loss of familiar reference points, (3) old needs that remain unmet, (4) new needs, and (5) old expectations that are no longer congruent with the changing situation. Schumacher and Meleis (1994) proposed four categories of transition in which nurses are involved: developmental, health/illness, situational, and organizational. Developmental transitions are those that reflect life cycle transitions, such as adolescence, parenthood, and aging. Spross, Clarke, & Beauregard (2000) consider developmental transitions to include any intrapersonally focused transition, including changes in life cycle, self-perception, motivation, expectations, or meaning. Health/illness transitions were described by Schumacher and Meleis primarily as illness related, ranging from adapting to a chronic illness to being discharged from the hospital to home.

Transitions can include modifying risk factors, adapting to a chronic illness, adapting to the physiological and psychological demands of pregnancy, and numerous other clinical phenomena. Some health/illness changes are self-limiting (e.g., the physiological changes of pregnancy), whereas others are long term or chronic, reversible or irreversible.

The APN is also aware of the possibility of multiple transitions occurring as a result of one salient transition. While eliciting information on the primary transition that led the client to seek care, the APN is attending to verbal, nonverbal, and intuitive cues to identify other transitions and meanings associated with the primary one. Attending to the possibility of multiple transitions enables the APN to tailor coaching to the individual's particular needs and concerns.

Outcomes of transitions proposed by Schumacher and Meleis (1994) included subjective well-being, role mastery, and well-being of relationships. Quality-of-care outcomes could also be used as indicators of successful transitions. When one considered the direct, individual effects of APN coaching, the most relevant outcomes are those that are patient related. These could be traditional or emerging clinical outcomes, such as morbidity; mortality; medical complications; comfort; functional, physiological, or mental status; stress level; coping strategies; quality of life; patient satisfaction; and caregiver burden (Kolcaba, 1992; Lang & Marek, 1992; Naylor, Munro, & Brooten, 1991; Peplau, 1994). This description of transitions as a focus for APN coaching underscores the need for, and the importance of, a holistic orientation when helping individuals address their health and illness concerns.

Expert Coaching

Several assumptions that underlie the APNs' coaching and guiding must be made explicit. First, the entire discussion of coaching assumes the integration of the client's significant other or the client's proxy as appropriate. Second, although technical competence and clinical competence may be sufficient to teach a task, they are insufficient to coach patients through transitions. For example, persons with diabetes may be taught how to monitor their blood sugar and administer insulin with technical accuracy, but, if the impact of the transition from health to chronic illness that requires major lifestyle changes is not evaluated, then coaching and guidance cannot occur. Failure to assess the need for coaching when teaching patients about health and illness may influence the outcomes of individual and group teaching approaches. Third, the APN's skill as an expert coach and guide depends on a combination of clinical experience with a particular population and graduate education. The clinical and didactic content of graduate education extends the APN's repertoire of assessment skills, technical skills, interpersonal behaviors, and self-reflection abilities, enabling the APN to coach in situations that are broader in scope or more complex in nature. APNs also are able to be more explicit about the processes and outcomes of coaching.

Finally, the basis for expert APN coaching is the interaction of interpersonal, technical, and clinical competence with self-reflection. Expert coaching requires that APNs be self-aware and self-reflective as an interpersonal transaction is unfolding, so that they can shape communications and behaviors to maximize the therapeutic and educational goals of the clinical encounter. The ability to self-reflect and focus on the process of coaching as it is occurring implies that APNs are capable of the simultaneous execution of other skills. While interacting with a client, APNs integrate physical, cognitive, and intuitive skills such as physical examination, interviewing, attending to their own noncognitive reactions and those of the client, and interpreting these multiple sources of information. One might compare this process to the simultaneous translation of a speech into several languages as it is being given. The difference is that the simultaneous translations are being carried out by a single APN, not several translators.

Technical and clinical competence are well-defined aspects of established APN roles, and their importance to coaching cannot be overestimated. The evolution of specialties in advanced nursing practice has focused on defining and describing the technical and clinical skills required for advanced practice with particular populations. An important part of clinical competence is clinical experience with the populations that are the APN's focus. Ongoing development of the APN's coaching competency depends on applying self-reflection to clinical experiences in order to acquire new coaching knowledge and skills that cannot be found in any textbook.

Establishing a caring, therapeutic relationship with a client demands that the APN be emotionally responsive, not distant. The nurse and patient enter the relationship as whole persons, complete with talents, goals, needs, and wishes, but the focus of the interpersonal process is on addressing the patient's potentials and goals (Martocchio, 1987; Montgomery, 1993).

Coaching Assessment, Processes, and Outcomes

Patient assessment is the basis of determining which interventions will be used. Assessments have two purposes: (1) establishing and building a relationship and (2) collecting data. Assessment entails getting to know the patient as a person and learning the patient's pattern of responses, including habits, practices, preferences, usual demeanor, and self-presentation (Jenny & Logan, 1992). Assessment must extend beyond the individuals to consider the clients' communities and social mileu, because social and contextual variables often influence the APN's ability to provide effective care. Both the APN's and the patient's cultural and political location powerfully influence their understandings of health, illness, language, identity, social roles, and historical issues.

In addition to getting to know the patient and using strategic communication, APNs use their observations of themselves, the patients, and the interactive process to decode patient's behaviors and the content of their communications for significance (Kasch & Dine, 1988). They need to grasp the patient's perspective, including salient aspects of the patient's self-definition (Olesen et al., 1990). This understanding is critical for selecting coaching behaviors to help people who need to make lifestyle changes, reduce risk, or manage chronic illness.

Cognitive variables such as knowledge, self-care skills, motivation, coping style, habitual stressors, and personal preferences for control affect people's experience of and ability to accept, adjust to, or adapt to transitional experiences (Brooten et al., 1991; Corbin & Strauss, 1992; Jenny & Logan, 1992; Kasch & Dine, 1988; Schumachaer & Meleis, 1994). The environment, including resources, relationship, social support, setting of care, and contextual variables, can mediate transitions (Brooten et al., 1991; Corbin & Strauss, 1992; Schumacher & Meleis, 1994). Role demands and responsibilites that may interfere with therapeutic self-care need to be identified (Connelly, 1993). Level of planning, including problem and need identification, organization of phase-related interventions, and communication, influences the success of the transition. Physical and emotional well-being also determine how the transition process is experienced (Schumacher & Meleis, 1994). The nature of the health concern; the degree of symptomatology, perceived vulnerability, and seriousness; and the degree of predictability or certainty about one's experience of the body can make for smooth or chaotic transitions.

Process and Outcomes

Coaching processes used by APNs focus on fostering involvement, choice, and independence. In coaching a patient, APNs have four main tasks: 1) interpreting unfamiliar diagnostic and treatment demands, 2) coaching the patient through alienated stances (e.g., anger and hopelessness), 3) identifying changing relevance as demands or symptoms of the illness change, and 4) ensuring that cure is enhanced by care. Both processes and outcomes can be categorized by focus: bodily or physical, affective/interpersonal/spiritual, cognitive/behavioral, and social.

APNs attend to issues of timing and sequencing in teaching and counseling patients. Knowing the patient enables APNs to take risks, adopt stances that are unusual or unpopular, and make the system work in order to shape patients' transitional experiences, a quality of APN direct care that has been described as "fearlessness" (Koetters, 1989).

Development of APN's Coaching Competence

Becoming an expert coach requires a combination of education, experience, interpersonal competence, and self-reflection on one's practice. Although scientific and technical knowledge are essential for effective coaching, it is in the coaching of clients that the art of advanced nursing practice is fully expressed. APNs need a highly refined range of interpersonal skills to coach people through multifaceted transitions. The strategies used to develop coaching expertise are designed to groom reflective practice and a person-oriented interactive style. These are foundational abilities that APNs must develop to become skilled coaches.

Issues

Numerous factors in contemporary health care have increased the focus on patient education as a means of improving effectiveness and efficacy and achieving cost and quality outcomes. The emphasis in managed care on risk reduction (Harris, 1997), disease management (Weiss, 1998), and implementation of evidence-based practices requires that nurses establish partnerships with patients so that they can coach them in self-care and tailor interventions to the needs of the patient and the situational context.

One of the problems in discerning the impact of APN education on patient care is the inconsistency with which the "nurse or APN dose" of the intervention is described. If patient education is effective and if efficient patient education is one of the solutions to reducing the costs of health care, more needs to be understood about the process of patient teaching used by APNs and how it promotes adherence to therapies and self-care.

An important consideration in implementing the APN coaching and guidance competency is the extent of health illiteracy in the United States. Literacy is defined as "an individual's ability to read, write, and speak in English, and compute and solve problems at levels of proficiency necessary to function on the job and in society, to achieve one's goals, and develop one's knowledge and potential" (1991 National Literacy Act passed by the U.S. Congress and cited in Ad Hoc Committee on Health Literacy for the Council on Scientific Affairs, American Medical Association, 1999, p. 552). The National Adult Literacy Survey revealed that nearly one quarter of the U.S. population (40 to 44 million people) are functionally illiterate. The large number of individuals with marginal literacy skills (about 50 million) means that about one half of adults in this country have reading and computational skills that are inadequate to meet the demands of daily life (Kirsch et al., 1993).

APNs coach patients through transitions. In the APN, graduate education and technical, clinical, and interpersonal competence interact with self-reflection to produce a diverse set of coaching skills and the ability to invent new coaching processes in the midst of novel clinical encounters. This is an extremely complex skill that relies on APNs' human and professional qualities. Although coaching processes occur simultaneously, they are not automatic. APNs can usually describe the intent of coaching interventions and explain their selection of one approach over another. What may seem automatic is actually very deliberate; the APN has learned what has worked in similar encounters and uses it over and over. In using a person-centered style with a patient, the APN remains open to cues that the approach may not work in this particular encounter, thereby remaining flexible and aware of alternatives. The ability to coach patients depends on direct care experiences in which new human responses, possibilities for growth, and new coaching strategies are revealed through APNs' encounters with patients and families as they experience health and illness and new technologies and new therapies.

Consultant

Consultation is a role utilized by APNs to offer their own clinical expertise to other colleagues or to seek additional information to enhance their own practice. It has the potential to increase the APNs ability and skill in providing expert nursing care. Consultation is distinguished from supervision, collaboration, referral, and co-management. These terms continue to be used interchangeably in practice without clear distinctions. Each term suggests very distinct relationships and responsibilities.

In CNS roles, consultation is primarily directed toward staff nurses as a way of directly or indirectly influencing patient care. Although CNSs might serve as consultants to physicians and other clinicians, staff nurses and their patients are the primary focus. APNs need to be clear and articulate about the implications of such terms such as "collaboration," "supervision," "direction," and "consultation". Medical societies may use such terminology with a clear intent to mandate hierarchal relationships with physicians in order to limit APN practice. Because mandated relationships between APNs and physicians may constrain the APN consultation role, it is important that APNs be aware of the statues and norms that regulate their practices.

Through consultation, APNs create networks with other APNs, physicians, and other colleagues, offering and receiving advice and information that can improve patient care and one's clinical knowledge and skills. Consultation also can help to shape and develop the practices of consultees and protégés, thereby indirectly but not significantly improving the quality, depth, and comprehensiveness of care available to populations of patients and families. Consultation offers APNs the opportunity to positively influence health care outcomes beyond the direct patient care encounter.

Distinguishing Consultation from Co-Management, Referral, and Collaboration

The primary characteristic that distinguishes consultation from co-management, referral, and supervision is the degree to which one assumes responsibility for the direct clinical management of a problem that falls within one's area of expertise. *Consultation* is an interaction between two professionals in which the consultant is recognized as having specialized expertise (Caplan 1970; Caplan & Caplan, 1993). *Co-management* is the process whereby one professional manages some aspects of a patient's care while another professional manages other aspects of the same patient's care. *Referral*, another frequently encountered term, describes a situation in which the clinician making the referral relinquishes responsibility for care (or aspects of care), either temporarily or permanently. *Collaboration* is a process that underlies the professional interactions involved in consultation, co-management, referral, and supervision. Therefore the discussion of consultation assumes collaboration as essential to the process.

Distinguishing Consultation from Clinical and Administrative Supervision

There are characteristics of supervision that distinguish it from consultation, and it is important that the supervisor and supervisee understand that supervision is different from consultation. The term "clinical supervision," as used in mental health, describes an ongoing supportive and educational process between a more senior and expert clinician and a less senior, more novice clinician. The goals of clinical supervision are to develop the knowledge, skills, self-esteem, and autonomy of the supervisee (Caplan & Caplan, 1993). Unlike the consultant, the supervisor generally is responsible for safeguarding the care of the supervisee's patients and is accountable in that respect for the work of the supervisee (Caplan & Caplan, 1993). Also unlike the consultant, who is often an outsider to the organization or unit where the consultation occurs, the supervisor and supervisee commonly are employed by the same organization and work together in the same clinical area. The supervisor and supervisee generally are in hierarchical positions with the supervisor being in a higher position (Caplan & Caplan, 1993). Although the ultimate goal of supervision and consultation are the same, namely, assisting another professional to enhance knowledge, skills, and abilities as they care for patients and families, the processes, relationships, and responsibilities are different.

Types of Consultation

There are four different types of consultation (Caplan, 1970). *Client-centered case consultation* is the most common type of consultation. The primary goal of this type of consultation is assisting the consultee to develop an effective plan of care for a patient who has a particularly difficult or complex problem. In client-centered case consultation, the consultant often sees the patient directly to complete an assessment of the patient and to make a recommendation to the consultee for the consultee's management of the case. This is often a one-time evaluation, although sometimes a follow-up by the consultant is needed. A positive experience with handling the specific case will enhance the consultee's ability so that future patients with similar problems can be managed more effectively.

In *consultee-centered case consultation,* improving patient care is important, but the emphasis is focused directly on the consultee's problem in handling the situation. Thus, the primary goal is to assist the consultee to acquire the knowledge, skill, confidence, or objectivity needed to address the problem effectively. In consultee-centered case consultation, the task for the consultant is to understand and remedy the problems of the consultee in managing a particular case. Usual problems, as noted, are lack of knowledge, skill, confidence, or objectivity.

The consultant may educate the consultee further on the issues presented by the patient or may suggest alternative strategies for dealing with the problem. This is probably the most common type of consultation sought by APNs. The consultant may seek to bolster the confidence of the consultee in handling the problem, if in the opinion of the consultant the consultee has the ability and potential to do so. If the problem presented by the consultee is a lack of processional objectivity, the consultant can help the consultee to identify the factors interfering with the consultee's ability to see the patient realistically. It may be that the difficulties in some way mirror or symbolize the consultee's personal difficulties and cloud the consultee's ability to see the reality of the situation. Effective consultation can foster orderly reflection and extend the frames of reference used by the consultee to solve the problems (Caplan & Caplan, 1993). Both client-centered and consultee-centered case consultations have been important activities in traditional CNS practice.

Program-centered administrative consultation focuses on the planning and administration of clinical services. *Consultee-centered administrative consultation* focuses on the consultee's (or group of consultees') difficulties as they interfere with the organization's objectives. APNs many be involved in all four types of consultation at various times.

Principals of Consultation

The following principles of consultation are derived from the field of mental health (Caplan, 1970; Caplan & Caplan, 1993; Lipowski, 1981):

1. The consultation is usually initiated by the consultee
2. The relationship between the consultant and consultee is nonhierarchical and collaborative
3. The consultant always considers contextual factors when responding to the quest for consultation
4. The consultant has no direct authority for managing patient care
5. The consultant does not prescribe but makes recommendations
6. The consultee is free to accept or reject the recommendation of the consultant
7. The consultation should be documented

Consultants should be aware that the purposes for which they have been consulted may change or expand during the process of consulting. Often, APN consultants accomplish several purposes at once. Over the course of the consultation, being explicit about the goal or outcome of the consultation is essential if APNs are to evaluate the impact of consultation on practice.

The Consultation Process

Assessment of the consultation problem begins with evaluation of the request itself. An important component of assessment is to confirm with the consultee that consultation is, in fact, the appropriate strategy for addressing the problem (rather than a referral, for example). At this stage, it is possible that the consultant and consultee decide that an alternative process is needed (e.g., shifting to co-management or referral). The consultant confirms that the problem has been accurately identified and falls within the realm of the consultant's expertise, and clarifies the nonhierarchical nature of the relationship between the consultant and consultee. The consultant also confirms that the consultee will remain clinically responsible for the patient who is the focus of the consultation. The consultant must remember that the consultee is ultimately free to accept of reject her or his recommendations. Once the request itself has been considered, the consultant gathers information from the consultee about the specific nature of the problem. The consultant tries to determine whether the patient has unusually difficult and complex problems (patient-centered consultation) and whether the problem results from the consultee's lack of knowledge, skill, confidence, or objectivity (consultee-centered consultation). Once the request, the nature of the relationship, and appropriateness of consultation have been established, the consultant focuses on gathering data related to the consultation problem. This may include direct assessment of the patient. The consultant also considers the ecological field of the consultation, which includes the systems and contexts that may influence the patient and family, the consultee and staff, and the setting in which the consultation takes place.

The consultant uses available resources such as patient records, direct assessment of the patient, and interviews with staff to *identify the exact problem* or problems that are to be the focus of the consultation. This may or may not be the one for which help was sought. Some consultation problems are simple and do not require extensive data collection. Others are complex and may require extensive chart review for a longstanding problem or calls to referring clinicians when incomplete data have been provided. The consultant shares the identified problem and validates it with the consultee. Since the problem frequently includes a lack of expertise on the part of the consultee, the consultant will want to use tact as the problem is identified and discussed. Interpersonal qualities of the consultant are crucial and are discussed later.

Once the specific problem or problems have been identified, the consultant and consultee *consider interventions* that will address the problem(s). The consultant may intervene directly with the consultee using such approaches as education, assisting with reinterpretation of the problem, or identification of appropriate resources if the problem is the consultee's lack of experience with the problem. If the problem results from a particularly difficult patient situation, the consultant may assist with the process of clinical decision making by providing alternative perspectives on the problem and recommending specific interventions. It may be that more data are needed to further analyze the situation and a decision needs to be made about whether the consultee or the consultant will gather more data. If the consultee accepts the recommendations of the consultant, together they negotiate how the interventions will be carried out and by whom. If the consultant is to intervene directly with the patient, the consultee must understand her or his ongoing responsibility for the patient and agree to the consultant's interventions. Together they identify additional resources and determine the time frame for the consultation (one time or ongoing).

Following the intervention, the consultant and consultee engage in *evaluation*. Evaluating the success or lack of success of the intervention and the overall consultation is essential to the consultation process. It the problem is resolved, evaluation offers an opportunity for review, confirmation of the enhanced effectiveness of the consultee in managing the problem (underscoring the new skills and abilities or understanding of the situation by the consultee), and closure. If problems remain, reassessment offers the consultant and consultee another opportunity for problem solving.

Characteristics of the APN Consultant

Self-awareness and interpersonal skills are essential for the consultant (Barron, 1989; Barron & White, 1996). For a model of consultative practice to be implemented, it is critical that APNs first value themselves and the specialized expertise they have developed. One must appreciate one's skills and knowledge before the possibilities for consultation can be envisioned.

A good consultant must be able to suspend judgment and avoid stereotyping. When consultation is sought, often what is needed is a fresh perspective. Self-understanding allows the consultant to see consultation issues realistically and without prejudice. It is not uncommon for a consultant to step into a highly emotionally charged situation. Self-awareness, understanding, and being able to remain centered and self-possessed are key to remaining objective and clear. It can be meaningful and helpful for the consultant to have a trusted colleague or supervisor with whom to share and review consultation situations.

It is also important that the consultant be able to establish warm, respectful, and accepting relationships with consultees. The initiation of a consultation request often is associated with a sense of vulnerability on the part of the consultee, who recognizes that assistance is required to help manage the situation at hand. The consultant must also communicate confidence in the consultee's ability to overcome the difficulties resulting in the consultation request. When the consulant creates a climate of trust and acceptance, the consultee can then be willing to risk vulnerability and genuineness with the consultant.

Common Consultation Situations

Depending on one's particular APN role, certain consultation situations may be more common than others. Patient- and consultee-centered case consultations are the most common requests APNs are likely to get.

APN-APN Consultation

Within one's specialty or agency, APNs may take for granted the available APN consulting resources. They may not think of their interactions about patient care as consultation because they occur in the hallway or over coffee. Consultation among APNs may be more or less formal depending on the culture of the unit or clinic, the relationships among the APNs, and the specialty populations seen in the facility. Norwood (1998) discussed the importance of, and practicalities related to APNs seeking consultation from other APNs. She noted that APNs readily think of themselves as consultants but may overlook opportunities for seeking consultation. She outlined the following factors as relevant when considering the use of a consultant: cost savings, objectivity, politics, when not to seek consultation, and issues to consider when choosing a consultant.

APN-Physician Consultation

When consulting with other APNs or physicians, an APN is likely to be fairly far along in the problem-solving process. The need for consultation is often related to the consultee's level of diagnostic uncertainty (Colman, 1992). Experienced APNs often have a clear definition of the problem and a preliminary plan to address it that they wish to validate or reformulate, depending on the consultant's advice. APN-APN or APN-physician consultation is sophisticated and high-level. When a hierarchical relationship exists between an APN and a physician, the APN who consults with a physician may defer to the physician's decisions, downplaying or ignoring first-hand knowledge of the patient. However, numerous descriptions of successful collaborative practices between physicians and APNs exist (Barron & White, 1996). Such practices embrace the nonhierarchical relationship we believe is key to effective consultation. There are APN-physician exchanges where true consultation occurs; however, much of the language that defines relationships between APNs and physicians involve the terms "co-management," "referral," and "supervision." Consultation between APNs and physicians can highlight for each what APNs know – that is, a deep appreciation for the human responses related to health and illness – and what physicians know, a deep understanding of disease and treatment. When both areas of expertise are available to patients and their families, truly holistic, comprehensive, and individualized care is offered.

APN-Staff Nurse Consultation

Part of implementing consultation means teaching staff how and when to consult. In the early days, CNSs often engaged in active case-finding to identify the patients who needed the knowledge and skills they had, because CNSs were not "assigned" to patients and staff nurses. By building this kind of clinical caseload, they demonstrated to staff how consultation might be helpful. Of note, CNSs tended both to do direct consultation and to consult with other professionals to assist the staff with problem solving and enhancing patient care. Once relationships are established and staff perceive that the APN consultant is approachable, respectful, and helpful, then staff will initiate contact with the consultant when complex clinical issues arise.

Documentation and Legal Considerations

Although it has been stressed that the consultee remains clinically responsible for the patient who is the focus of the consultation, it is also critical to appreciate that APN consultants are also accountable for their practices relative to the consultation problem. The overall responsibilities of the consultant are gathering accurate data about the consultation problem, making reasonable recommendations, and giving good advice. Consultants who are working within the same organization as the consultees have a higher degree of accountability in relation to the patient care situations for which they are consulted than do consultants who come from outside the organization. APNs who are consulting should, therefore, know the organizational structure well and be certain that the APN consultation responsibilities are consistent with the overall job description of the APN.

APNs must be cognizant of their responsibility to adhere to the standard of practice for their specialty areas in all aspects of practice, including consultation. A nurse-patient relationship exists when the consultation sees the patient directly, receives payment for the consultation, or becomes aware of gross negligence in clinical care.

The consultant's assessment of the problem and recommendations for clinical problem solving should be clearly articulated in the documentation. When the patient is not seen directly, the consultant will want to decide whether or not it is appropriate to document the consultation in the patient's record. If the primary focus of the consultation is on education of the consultee in relation to the consultation problem, documentation in the patient's chart is not necessary.

Developing the Practice of Consultation

An outcome of nursing consultation, especially consultation over time, is to enhance the professional development and practice of nurse consultees. Consultation can clearly enhance the clinical knowledge and practice of nurses requesting consultation. A goal for consultation is to enable the consultee to manage future similar situations effectively. Evaluation of the consultation itself with the consultee is enormously important. It can enhance the learning and skill of both the consultee and the consultant.

Initially, consultants must market their services to potential consultees. Setting, niche identification, workload, and experience are all issues that contribute to the time and focus an APN may have for consultation efforts. Over time, staff and colleagues recognize the APN's skill, and the APN may need to develop strategies to deal with large numbers of requests. Setting priorities and identifying alternative resources are important activities, as the consultation practice becomes more and more recognized and valued.

Consultation has the potential to influence patient care both directly and beyond the direct care encounter. Consultation offers APNs the opportunity to both share and receive the clinical expertise necessary to meet the increasingly challenging and diverse demands of patient care.

Researcher

The role of researcher has long been considered integral to the practice of clinical nurse specialists (Hodgman 1983; McGuire & Harwood, 1989) and reflects the critical contribution they have made to nursing knowledge and to scientifically-based practice. The foundation of APN research competencies consists in part of two related concepts: (1) research utilization (using research in practice) (Stetler, 1985), and (2) evidence-based medicine (basing practice on systematic scientific observation, with controlled randomized clinical trials providing the strongest levels of evidence) (Evidence-Based Working Group, 1992). A set of research competencies for APNs ranging from basic activities (e.g., appraising scientific literature) to advanced activities (e.g., developing institutional mechanisms for incorporating research into practice) should be evident.

Research Competencies

A research role for CNSs consists of three levels of research involvement: (1) activities related to identifying researchable problems, enhancing the clinical relevance of research, and facilitating the use of research by nurses and others in the clinical setting; (2) activities using the research process to conduct quality improvement, replication, case study, and secondary analysis studies; and (3) activities related to conducting independent or collaborative research. The levels of CNS research involvement evolved into three research competencies (McGuire & Harwood, 1996): (I) interpretation and use of research, (II) evaluation of practice, and (III) conducting research within a collaborative context. The use of integrative reviews of research by APNs as a basis for making decisions about nursing actions and interventions is an example of the research utilization competencies for APNs and is a key component of evidence-based practice (Stetler, Morsi, et al., 1998). Information taken from such reviews can be combined with other data to develop effective protocols for integrating scientific evidence into clinical care and changing clinical outcomes.

OVERVIEW OF RESEARCH COMPETENCIES AND LEVELS OF ACTIVITY		
COMPETENCY	BASIC LEVEL	ADVANCED LEVEL
I. Interpretation and use of research	• Incorporate relevant research findings appropriately into own practice • Assist others to incorporate research into individual or unit practice	• Develop programmatic and/or departmental research utilization process
II. Evaluation of practice	• Use existing individual and/or aggregate data to evaluate nursing practice • Collaborate in conduct of evaluation studies	• Identify and/or develop practice-specific package of outcome criteria • Lead the conduct of evaluation studies
III. Participation in collaborative research	• Identify research problems • Develop study procedures • Assist with recruitment • Participate in interventions • Identify nurse-sensitive outcomes • Collect outcomes data	

Interpretation and Use of Research

Interpreting and using existing research in practice constitute the focal point of this competency, which is based on the concepts of research utilization and evidence-based practice. At the heart of this research competency for APNs, is the critical appraisal of research for its scientific merit as well as its suitability/appropriateness for application to practice a given setting. A key component of evidence-based practice is the notion of "levels" (or strength) of evidence, which emanated originally from the Agency for Healthcare Quality and Research (AHRQ) clinical practice guidelines. Research utilization provides the means through which nursing or clinical science (the foundation of practice) is solidified, expanded, and actually used to guide or drive practice. That is, nurses read, evaluate, and use relevant research findings in order to improve the scope, content, and quality of their practice. These improved practices are then evaluated, and, if outcomes are positive, the value of the research on which they are based is substantiated, and the scientific foundation (science) of nursing practice is strengthened.

McGuire (1992) described research utilization as a complex process consisting of five essential components: (1) *dissemination/acquisition* of research findings to and by appropriate individuals and agencies, (2) *evaluation of merit and clinical applicability* of research findings, (3) *incorporation of research findings* into practice through various mechanisms, (4) *evaluation of research-based practice* through assessment of predetermined outcome parameters, and (5) *socialization* of nurses into the belief that research-based practice is not only desirable but necessary.

Skills needed for dissemination/acquisition include being able to identify literature databases and other resources and to find and retrieve literature. Of particular importance to APNs in all specialty areas is the ability to identify existing clinical guidelines based on research. The authors of such guidelines have already undertaken the task of identifying, retrieving, reviewing, and synthesizing available research and clinical information in order to apply it to practice.

Evaluation of Practice

The second research competency, evaluating advanced nursing practice that results from implementation of research-based practice, is conceptualized as encompassing the process that individual APNs (or groups of APNs) can use to evaluate aspects of their practice. It is important to distinguish it from outcomes research, outcomes measurement (Deaton, 1998a, 1998b), or the broader based studies of advanced nursing practice outcomes. The first component of practice evaluation involves selection of appropriate criteria and outcome measures, which are highly specific to the practice being evaluated. It is important to match these criteria and outcome measures to the interventions being employed. Multiple studies have examined outcomes in groups of patients receiving care from an APN. Others have compared outcomes of APN care versus that of other care providers. Although such studies have been important to establishing the cost-effectiveness of various APN specialties, they leave many questions unanswered regarding the specific APN interventions that contribute to favorable outcomes, as well as the "dose" of intervention needed (Brooten & Naylor, 1995). Specific APN interventions require evaluation, as do nursing interventions that serve as nursing practice standards or norms. A variety of general outcome criteria can be selected, such as length of stay, number of clinic visits, readmission rates, overall cost of care, patient satisfaction, and many others. Selection of specific parameters relevant to the individual APN's practice may be more appropriate.

Participation in Collaborative Research

The third research competency involves participation in collaborative nursing or interdisciplinary research studies conducted to generate knowledge that defines optimal nursing or other interventions for particular populations and specific clinical problems (Brooten & Naylor, 1995). A more realistic competency, APN's participation in collaborative research is usually highly context-driven. There is a need to make research a priority, to collaborate with others, to break projects into manageable parts, to structure work for multiple outcomes, and to garner the necessary resources. The APN, regardless or type of practice or setting, is the most likely individual to understand the clinical issues and questions in a given patient population. This individual can identify nursing practice problems and work collaboratively as a consultant with academically-based researchers to translate these problems into researchable questions and work with the research team in identifying nurse-sensitive outcomes. The APN can also be involved in helping to develop methods or study procedures that not only are clinically feasible but help minimize burden to staff and patients. Such collaboration can significantly enhance the clinical relevance and quality of research (McGuire & Harwood, 1989) as well as enhance its scientific rigor (McGuire, et al., 2000). Another viable collaborative activity is to assist researchers with identification and recruitment of appropriate subjects for a study. Participation in collaborative research is an important competency for APNs, although clearly less critical to the quality and effectiveness of their own practices than are interpretation and use of research, and evaluation of practice.

Current Trends

Changes in health care delivery have affected the research competencies needed by APNs, who play a significant role in defining research-based standards of care for specific patient populations, in evaluating the outcomes of such standards in individuals and groups, and in working with others on collaborative research to establish appropriate health care practices. APNs will need research competencies to help them determine the best care, appropriate resources, and feasible outcome evaluation mechanisms (Spross & Heaney, 2000). Through research competencies, APNs can demonstrate the value of their practice in producing better patient outcomes, be they quality of life, safety, satisfaction, or financial outcomes. In a collaborative practice setting, the APN is ideally positioned to promote research utilization or evidence-based practice in areas that physicians have traditionally not addressed, such as symptom management or health promotion.

Research suggests that there are many areas in which health care provided by APNs may result in better outcomes at lower cost than care provided by physicians or, when APNs and physicians have the same authority and responsibilities, equivalent outcomes (Mundinger et al., 2000). The future of advanced nursing practice, in its preferred state of collaborative rather than supervised surrogate practice, hinges on research in all its manifestations – that is, interpretation and use of research, evaluation of outcomes of advanced nursing practice, and knowledge building through participation in the conduct of theory-based research. This future of advanced nursing practice also depends not only on demonstration of positive cost and quality outcomes for patients managed by APNs but on a definition of specific components of nursing practice that lead to positive outcomes. APNs are expected to integrate clinical expertise and specific research competencies to improve the care of their patients and to provide clinical leadership for other nurses (Cronenwett, 1995). The development of appropriate clinical practice guidelines depends on a process of critically evaluating research findings and determining their applicability to practice, activities that are clearly within the scope of APNs' practice skills and qualifications (McGuire & Harwood, 1989, 1996; Stetler & diMaggio, 1991).

An increasing emphasis on interdisciplinary approaches to care also is driving efforts to provide research-based practice. Tools used to manage patients include critical pathways, algorithms, and other structured approaches to managing specific patient populations or problems. Interdisciplinary plans of care incorporate mechanisms for care documentation and for tracking and analyzing outcome data. APNs often provide leadership in the development of these approaches (Lindeke & Block, 1998), particularly when they function as case managers. These activities provide opportunities to use nursing research, to incorporate the services and interventions of APNs into care delivery systems, and to advocate for holistic care of patients and families. Without adequate preparation in research competencies, APNs may find it difficult to assume these responsibilities. In addition to using research findings, there is a need to demonstrate through the research process that positive patient outcomes result from APNs' interventions (Brooten & Naylor, 1995). When APNs' interventions are judged effective through systematic research, they should be included in interdisciplinary and nursing standards of care.

Key APN Competencies as used by Clinical Nurse Specialists 3

Clinical Leader

Leadership is a core competency of the APN. Leadership models that empower followers, include others outside of nursing, and allow for change to occur seem to "fit" the best in these unsettled times.

Useful Leadership Definitions and Models

Burns (1978) defined *transactional leadership* as occurring when one person takes the initiative to foster the exchange of something of value, either economic, psychological, or political, to another person. The leader and follower may have related purposes but are not necessarily connected by common goals. Leaders incite, stimulate, share with, pacify, and satisfy their followers in an interdependent, interactional exchange. *Transformational leadership* is a process whereby change occurs in which "the purposes of the leader and follower become fused, creating unity, wholeness and a collective purpose" (p. 83). The *situational* approach to leadership suggests that leadership is situationally dependent, with identified leaders and followers in interchangeable roles based on environmental demands. *Roving leadership* is a participatory process that legitimizes the situational leadership of empowered followers through the support and approval of a hierarchical leader.

APNs will assume both leader and follower roles, and need to develop skills to know when these different roles are indicated, and when the situation warrants their moving from follower to leader. The APN as a leader who has a vision of collaboration among health care team members may facilitate an atmosphere that supports individuals (followers) in assuming the leadership role in various situations. The APN does not cease being the leader by empowering colleagues to appropriately assume a leadership role. In fact, this important approach may be an effective way of both sharing a vision and sharing a power. Good leaders are constantly striving to become better, to empower others, and to facilitate change.

Types of Leadership

Certain situations require distinct types of leadership that allow leadership styles to emerge in several unique forms and settings. *Clinical leadership* occurs when APNs learn with and from others about how to build appropriate working relationships with health team members, how to instill confidence in patients and colleagues, and how to problem solve as part of a team (Warden, 1997). Clinical leaders are role models and mentors who empower patients and colleagues. They serve as change agents who implement change strategies that improve patient care and enhance APN practice enactment. *Entrepreneurial leadership* refers to those APN leaders who go outside of traditional employment systems to create new opportunities to exercise their special abilities (Ballien, 1998). *Organizational leadership* refers to situations in which leaders are formally elected or appointed to positions of power within defined organizations and groups.

The Process of Change

Subsumed within the competency of leadership for APNs is the competency of being a change agent. Being a successful change agent requires many of the skills and attributes that are needed to be a successful APN leader. However, it is important to understand the complex concepts and forces that drive the health care system, and how APNs take on the important activity of change agentry every time they enact leadership (Klein, Gabelnick, & Herr, 1998). Change occurs at both the system and the personal level, and Covey (1989) proposed that one must deal with core values to successfully change or serve as an agent of change.

Driving and Restraining Forces of Change

Traditional models of the change process are insufficient for addressing change today because these models conceived of change as a linear process that occurred over time. Although they are less useful, certain concepts from these traditional models are still relevant. For example, Lewin's Force Field Analysis model is helpful in understanding the psychodynamics of change. He described a state of equilibrium between driving and restraining forces that encourage or discourage movement. It is the effect of these opposing forces that make change, especially rapid change, so difficult (Lewin, 1951). These external and internal forces or tensions also can be described as the cognitive dissonance (the conflict between actions and values) that may be evident during change and that cause the uncomfortable feelings that people undergoing change often experience. Driving and restraining forces are useful for APNs in terms of planning for change and evaluating both planned and unplanned changes as they unfold. An example is the movement toward multistate licensure that is gaining momentum as APN practice moves across state lines. Forces such as reimbursement and prescriptive authority can serve as both positive and negative influences for APNs as this new form of regulation develops.

Planned Versus Unplanned Change

The Big Three Model developed by Kantor, Stein, and Jick (1992), and the changes processes described by Lewin (1951) and Bridges (1991), all depend on a planned evolution for change that allows for time to work through or bridge the changes over a trajectory that allows for ending of the old order, education to the new order, and then a restructuring of the new version. Planned change models are helpful in settings where time is not a factor and are useful in helping the APN leader to frame a positive evolution to a new structure for care in certain settings. Unplanned and constant change is the reality of today's health care environment. Leaders need to understand the personal implications of change if the culture of change is to be realized. APNs with highly developed psychosocial skills are poised to be pivotal change agent leaders in this process.

Political Activism and Advocacy

The core elements that define contemporary leadership, such as shared vision, systems thinking, and the ability to engage in high-level communication within the context of a changing environment, are all basic to political interaction. There is little room for discussion about whether APNs need to take on the mantle of policy maker and patient advocate as part of their leadership role. For many, it falls within the context of a moral imperative.

Key Attributes of Successful APN Leaders

Personal Attributes

Several personal attributes are deemed necessary for successful leaders. These qualities are very broad and support the concept that all leadership today is required to be interdisciplinary. Personal attributes for APN leadership include:

- Vision, coupled with the ability to set priorities
- A good sense of timing
- Self-confidence, assertiveness, and the willingness to take risks
- Expert communication skills and the willingness to connect with others
- Boundary management
- Respect for cultural diversity
- Balance in personal and professional life
- Willingness to collaborate, change and negotiate, fail and begin again

Mentoring and Empowerment

Two major proficiencies, empowerment and mentoring, stand out as important skills in the process of leadership, change, and advocacy. The responsibility to empower and mentor is central to all of the definitions of leadership and change. The ability to help others to grow and to encourage them toward self-actualization requires competent, caring leaders who are interested in the success and well-being of their followers. Coaching and guiding with an awareness and attentiveness to the needs and concerns of followers are basic characteristics of successful leaders. Leading by example, role modeling, enabling followers, and encouraging them to move upward are all leadership aptitudes. Mentors have been defined by many as having those qualities that epitomize success in their own careers and the ability and desire to help others achieve success. The reward for the mentor is to step back and enjoy the success of the protégé who has succeeded in reaching the next level of competence.

Closely aligned to, but somewhat different from, the mentoring process is the process of empowerment. Empowerment is defined as giving power to another, enabling, giving authority. APNs operationalize this by enabling or giving power to other nurses, colleagues, and patients. Empowerment as a leadership strategy is guided by the shared vision of the leader and follower and a willingness of the leader to delegate power to others.

Acquiring Skills as APN Leaders, Change Agents, and Activists

A key attribute of APN leadership is the responsibility for cultural competence. The following levels of culturally competent leadership can be identified: (1) societal, (2) professional, (3) organizational, and (4) individual. For the APN, the responsibility for culturally competent care includes all four levels of the diversity system. Culturally competent care is care delivered with knowledge, sensitivity, and respect for the consumer/family's cultural/racial/ethnic background and reality.

Attributes of nurse leaders are:

- Expert communication skills
- Commitment
- Developing one's own style
- Risk taking
- Willingness to collaborate

Obstacles to Successful Leadership

There are several obstacles to achieving competence as an APN leader. Most of the obstacles result from conflict and/or competition between individuals or groups. Being respected rather than being "liked" is one desired criterion for leadership. Trying to "do it all" rather than delegating to others is a common trap that plagues busy leaders. Two other pitfalls include avoiding the direct confrontation of difficult issues and a lack of communication. One of the most important things that APNs do as leaders is to create community.

Collaborator

Collaboration can be thought of as one of several modes of interaction that occur between and among clinicians during the delivery of care. A variety of interactions can occur. These include parallel communication and functioning, information exchange, coordination, consultation, co-management, referral, and collaboration.

- *Parallel Communication*: Providers interact with a patient separately; they do not talk together before seeing a patient, nor do they see the patient together. There is no expectation of joint interactions.
- *Parallel Functioning*: Providers care for patients, addressing the same clinical problem, but do not engage in any joint or collaborative planning.
- *Information Exchange*: Informing may be one-or two-sided and may or may not require action or decision making. If action is needed, the decision is unilateral, not a result of joint planning.
- *Coordination*: The establishment of structures to minimize duplication of effort and to maximize efficient use of clients' and providers' resources.
- *Consultation*: The process whereby the clinician who is caring for a client seeks advice regarding a client concern but retains primary responsibility for care delivery.
- *Co-Management*: This refers to the process in which two or more clinicians provide care and each professional retains accountability and responsibility for defined aspects of care. This process usually arises from consultation in which a problem requires management that is outside the scope of practice of the referring clinician. One clinician usually retains responsibility for the majority of care (as in primary care settings) while the second provider is accountable for managing the problem that is outside the primary provider's expertise. Providers must be explicit with each other about their responsibilities.
- *Referral*: The process by which the APN directs the client to a physician or another practitioner for management of a particular problem or aspect of the client's care when the problem is beyond her or his expertise.

With the exceptions of parallel communication and parallel functioning, these processes require some level of interaction and communication among providers. Information exchange, coordination, consultation, co-management, and referral do not require collaboration as it is described here, although collaboration is likely to enhance them.

Collaboration requires individuals to interact holistically (sharing strengths, weaknesses, and emotions), to share power, and to remain open to the possibilities for personal and professional transformation that exist within a collaborative relationship. When the notions of shared values and commitment are included, it becomes clear that collaboration is a process that evolves over time. Collaboration describes relationships that are positive and work well for professionals and clients. There is room for disagreement in collaborative relationships; partners develop strategies for dealing with disagreement that are mutually satisfactory and enhance collaboration.

Collaboration Works

Collaboration is widely perceived as useful and desirable. Although there are few studies of collaboration that have measured patient outcomes systematically (Sullivan, 1998; Torres & Dominguez, 1998), both patient and provider benefits have been documented.

BENEFITS OF COLLABORATION

FOR PATIENTS	FOR PROVIDERS
• Improved quality of care	• Increased sharing of responsibility
• Increased patient satisfaction	• Increased sharing of expertise
• Lower mortality	• More mutually satisfying problem solving
• Improved patient outcomes	• Improved communications
• Patients feel more secure, cared for, closer to nurses	• Increased personal satisfaction
	• Increased quality of professional life
	• Enhanced mutual trust and respect
	• Bridges care-cure dichotomy
	• Expands horizons of providers
	• Avoids redundant care and ensures coverage
	• Empowers providers to influence health policy

Adapted from Sullivan, T.J. (1998). Collaboration: A health care imperative (pp. 26-27). New York: McGraw-Hill Health Professions Division; reprinted with permission.

The Effects of Failure to Collaborate

The failure to communicate and collaborate affects patients and clinician job satisfaction. Failure to collaborate may contribute to inefficiencies in patient care (Cooper, Henderson, & Dietrich, 1998; Grumbach & Coffman, 1998). Alpert, Goldman, Kilroy, and Pike (1992) found that job satisfaction and attitude were negatively affected when collaboration failed and that territoriality and competitiveness increased. However, the most important result of failure to collaborate is its negative effect on patient care.

Collaboration as an Ethical Issue and Institutional Imperative

Some writers have suggested that the failure to collaborate is an ethical issue. Compassionate, ethical patient care that provides a healing environment requires collaborative working relationships between physicians and nurses (Aroskar, 1998; Larson, 1999). Larson (1999) identified key beliefs about collaboration on which nurses and physicians differ: the importance of relationships, what constitutes effective and desirable communication, the degree to which communication and shared decision making occur, the authority nurses have to make decisions, and what strategies would improve communication. The failure to understand each other's perspectives, a prerequisite for collaboration, results in a difficult work environment and contributes to uncoordinated, unsafe care (Larson, 1999).

Gianakos (1997) identified three reasons for nurses and physicians to collaborate, and asserted that the ethical imperative to collaborate is the most important:

- Collaboration is a moral imperative - good patient care requires it
- Collaboration reinforces commitment to a common goal and reaffirms the message that patient welfare is the goal
- Collaboration enhances shared knowledge as physicians and nurses educate each other repeatedly about the patient

The evidence that collaboration works suggests that there are structural as well as interpersonal dimensions to collaboration. That is, although institutional policies or standards do not guarantee collaboration, they can establish expectations for communication and collaboration. Pellegrino (1996) concluded that human organization and relationships are more important than our mutual concerns over resources and technologies. The mutual goal of good patient care and the ethical imperative to collaborate should be at the center of any interdisciplinary effort to plan care or resolve conflicts in approaches to care.

Opportunities for Collaboration

There are numerous incentives for nurses, physicians, and other providers to collaborate. APNs, physicians, and other providers share a common purpose – the desire to provide good patient care. This mutual goal should be enough to ensure that collaboration occurs consistently. Each group of clinicians has unique, complementary, and overlapping skills that benefit patients. Efforts to reduce costs of health care offer APNs and physicians a common goal toward which to work and opportunities for learning from each other. Accreditation activities offer another opportunity to build collaborative relationships. The move towards a more community-based, health promotion/disease prevention model of care is further creating new opportunities for collaborative practice (Simpson, 1998).

Regulatory Issues

Legislation and regulations have been barriers to the implementation of collaborative roles (Fagin, 1992; Inglis & Kjervik, 1993). Although major strides have been made in some states, statutes and regulations often support a hierarchical structure that impedes collaboration between nurses and physicians. Language that mandates the nature of APN-physician relationships can undermine collaborative practice. Using such language to regulate interprofessional relationships presents risks to professional autonomy and effective collaboration for APNs and physicians. Collaboration cannot be mandated; it is a process that develops over time.

Characteristics of Effective Collaboration

Steele's (1986) analysis of collaboration among NPs and physicians revealed several characteristics: mutual trust and respect, an understanding and acceptance of each other's disciplines, positive self-image, equivalent professional maturity arising from education and experience, recognition that the partners are not substitutes for each other, and a willingness to negotiate. Hughes and Mackenzie (1990) outlined four characteristics of NP-physician collaboration: collegiality, communication, goal sharing, and task interdependence. Based on a review of CNS and interdisciplinary literature, Spross (1989) described three essential elements of collaboration: a common purpose, diverse and complementary professional knowledge and skills, and effective communication processes. Although this is not an exhaustive summary of the literature on collaboration, it is clear that shared values, effective interpersonal communication, and organizational structures can promote productive alliance among clinicians and create environments in which collaboration is valued and practiced.

Other essential characteristics are a common purpose, clinical competence, interpersonal competence (or a willingness to learn), and trust. Other attributes, such as a sense of humor, respect, and valuing each other's knowledge and skills reflect the nature of collaboration as an interpersonal process.

Common Purpose

The notion that a common purpose must be the basis for collaboration is well supported in the literature (Alpert et al., 1992; Arslanian-Engoren, 1995; Spross, 1989). Collaboration involves a bond, a union, and a degree of patient caring that goes beyond a single approach to care and represents a synergistic alliance that maximizes the contributions of each participant (Evans, 1994).

Collaboration, by definition, implies that the participants are interdependent. Recognizing their interdependence, team members can combine their individual perceptions and skills to synthesize more complex and comprehensive care plans (Forbes & Fitzsimmons, 1993). Each member brings a particular set of skills and unique expertise to the table for a combined strength that cannot be matched by individuals working alone. Like other characteristics, the common purpose(s) that initially brought partners together may change over time.

Clinical Competence

Clinical competence is perhaps the most important characteristic underlying a successful collaborative experience among clinicians, for without it the trust and desire needed to work together are not possible. Trust and respect are built on the assurance that each member is able to carry out her or his role and function in a competent manner. When collaborating clinicians can rely on each other to be clinically competent, mutual trust and respect develops.

Interpersonal Competence

Interpersonal competence is the ability to communicate effectively with colleagues in a variety of situations, including uncomplicated, routine interactions, disagreements, value conflicts and stressful situations. After clinical competence, interpersonal competence may be the most important individual characteristic needed for APNs to establish collaborative relationships.

Trust

Implicit in discussions of collaboration is the presence of mutual trust, mutual respect, and personal integrity, qualities evinced in the nature of interactions between partners. The development of trust and respect depends on clinical competence. A central theme of the development of trust is sharing. Partners are guided by a shared vision of the possibilities inherent in collaboration; they believe in the value of collaboration, and they are committed to achieving the relationship's potential (Krumm, 1992; Nugent & Lambert, 1996). Collaboration also means sharing in planning, decision making, problem solving, goal setting, and assuming responsibility (Baggs & Schmitt, 1988).

Conclusion

Collaboration works. Research supports the premise that collaboration results in better patient outcomes, including patient satisfaction, and provides personal and professional satisfaction for clinicians. Advanced practice nurses (APNs) must have or acquire interpersonal communication skills and behaviors that make collaboration with a broad range of professionals and clients possible. Collaboration between health care providers is an essential component of effective patient care. It is important that any discussion of collaborative relationships address both intradisciplinary collaboration among nurses and interdisciplinary collaboration between nurses and members of other disciplines.

The presence or absence of collaborative relationships affects patient care. Clients assume that their health care providers communicate and collaborate effectively. However, client dissatisfaction with care, unsatisfactory clinical outcomes, and clinician frustration often can be traced to a failure to collaborate. The ability to collaborate is a core competency of advanced nursing practice (Brown, 1998). Collaboration depends on clinical and interpersonal expertise and an understanding of factors that can promote or impede efforts to establish collegial relationships. As pressures to change mount in response to ongoing health care reform, and as the proportion of nonphysician health professionals increases, interdisciplinary collaboration at educational, clinical, and institutional levels is essential (Lindeke & Block, 1998).

Patient Advocate

Because nurses have a unique relationship to the patient and family, the moral position of nursing in the health care arena is distinct. As the complexity of issues intensifies, the role of the APNbecomes particularly important in the identification, deliberation, and resolution of complicated and difficult value choices. It is a basic tenet of the central definition of advanced nursing practice that ethical decision-making skills are part of the core competencies of all APNs.

Characteristics of Ethical Dilemmas in Nursing

An ethical or moral dilemma occurs when two (or more) morally acceptable courses of action are present and to choose one prevents selecting another. Although the scope and nature of moral dilemmas experienced by nurses reflect the varied clinical settings in which they practice, three general themes emerge when examining ethical issues in nursing practice. First, most ethical dilemmas that occur in the health care setting are interdisciplinary in nature. Issues such as refusal of treatment, end-of-life decision making, cost containment, and confidentiality all have multidisciplinary elements interwoven in the dilemmas, and therefore an interdisciplinary approach is necessary for successful resolution of the issue. Health care professionals bring varied viewpoints and perspectives into discussions of ethical issues, and these differing positions can lead to creative and collaborative decision making. Thus an interdisciplinary theme is prevalent in both the presentation and resolution of ethical problems.

Clear communication is an essential prerequisite for informed and responsible decision making. In fact, some ethical disputes reflect inadequate communication rather than a difference in values (LaMear-Tucker & Friedson, 1997). Clear and definitive communication with patients and families will increase understanding, lead to more knowledgeable decision making, and may improve compliance with current therapies. Within the multidisciplinary health care team, discussions are most effective when members are accountable for presenting information in a precise and succinct manner. The skill of listening is just as crucial in effective communication as having proficient verbal skills. Listening involves recognizing and appreciating various perspectives. To listen well is to allow others the necessary time to form and present their thoughts and ideas. In this way, good communication may be an effective tool in preventing ethical dilemmas. Furthermore, when ethical dilemmas arise, effective communication skills are the key to negotiating and facilitating a resolution.

Nurses have numerous and, at times, competing obligations to various stakeholders within the health care and legal systems (Lynch, 1991; Saulo & Wagener, 1996). Ethical deliberation involves analyzing and dealing with the differing and opposing demands that occur. The general themes of interdisciplinary involvement, thoughtful communication and balancing multiple commitments are prevalent in most ethical dilemmas. Although these characteristics emerge as common elements, specific ethical issues may be unique to the specialty area and clinical setting in which the APN practices.

The issues of quality of life and symptom management traverse acute and nonacute health care settings (Calkins, 1993; Omeryet al., 1995; Solomon et al., 1993; Winters, Glass & Sakurai, 1993). Pain relief and symptom management become problematic for nurses when physicians are reluctant to acknowledge the patient's problem and/or pre-scribe adequate amounts of medication to alleviate the patient's pain and suffering (Turner, Marquis & Burman, 1996; Omery et al., 1995; Solomon et al., 1993). Chronic illness, symptom management, and quality-of-life issues often are central to the ethical dilemmas and conflicts that nurses experience in their relationships with patients and professional colleagues.

The arrival of managed care has significantly changed the traditional practice of de-livering health care. Managed care goals of reduced expenditures and services, in-creased efficiency, enhanced quality of life for patients, and improved treatment and care of patients often compete, creating conflict and tension between parties and among nurses, physicians, and employers with diverse goals (Rowdin, 1995).

Technological advances, such as the rapidly expanding field of genetics, will further challenge APNs in the near future. APNs will encounter this information in a variety of settings and may be faced with discussing the need for, and perhaps results of, predic-tive testing for genetic disorders. Issues such as inadvertent detection of nonpaternity, denial of reimbursement for genetic testing, loss of eligibility for insurance, and the po-tential for discrimination may surface as the use of genetic technology increases (Wil-liams & Lea, 1995). Because genetic information is crucially linked to the concepts of privacy and confidentiality and the availability of this information is increasing, it is in-evitable that APNs will encounter ethical dilemmas related to the use of genetic data.

The complexity of ethical issues in the current health care environment and inabil-ity to reach agreement among parties has resulted in participants seeking legal settle-ment. The APN must understand the relevance of current laws and regulations on clinical practice. It is important that APNs not comingle legal perspectives with ethical decision making.

APNs engage in research as principal investigators, co-investigators, or data collec-tors for clinical studies and trials. Regardless of the level of involvement, the APN must support the best interests of the patient and uphold the ethical concepts of informed consent and truthfulness. Patients must understand if the research is considered thera-peutic or nontherapeutic and that they may withdraw from the study at any time.

Ethical Decision-Making Competencies

At the APN level, ethical involvement follows and evolves from clinical expertise. Ethi-cal involvement requires APNs to extend beyond the technical demands of clinical practice. The core competency of ethical decision making for APNs can be organized into three phases. Each phase relies on the acquisition of the knowledge and skills em-bedded in the previous level. These phases utilize the expert practice domains of moni-toring and ensuring the quality of health care practices, teaching/coaching functions, and the consulting role of the nurse (Fenton & Brykczynski, 1993).

PHASES OF DEVELOPMENT OF CORE COMPETENCY FOR ETHICAL DECISION MAKING		
	KNOWLEDGE	SKILL
Phase 1: Knowledge Development	Ethical theories Professional code Professional standards	Sensitivity to the ethical dimensions of clinical problems Evaluate practice setting for congruence with literature Identify ethical issues in the practice setting and bring to the attention of other team members Gather relevant literature related to problems identified
Phase 2: Knowledge Application – Moral Action	Ethical decision-making theories Mediation/facilitation strategies	Apply ethical decision-making theory to clinical problems Facilitate decision making using select strategies
Phase 3: Creating an Ethical Environment	Preventive ethics Minimizing barriers to ethical practice	Role-modeling, mentoring others Address barriers to ethical practice through system changes

Phase 1: Knowledge Development–Moral Action

The first phase in the ethical decision-making core competency is developing core knowledge in both ethical theories and principles and the ethical issues common to specific patient populations or clinical settings. A general understanding of ethical theories, principles, and rules is necessary to define and discern the essential elements of an ethical dilemma. A key aspect of this phase is developing the ability to distinguish a true ethical dilemma from a clinically problematic situation. The core knowledge of ethical theories should be tempered with an understanding of issues central to the patient populations with whom the APN works. As APNs assume positions in specific clinical areas or with particular patient populations, it is incumbent upon them to gain an understanding of the applicable laws, standards, and regulations, as well as relevant paradigm cases. The emphasis in this stage is on cognitive mastery, in which the APN learns the theories, principles, rules, paradigm cases, and relevant laws that influence ethical decision making.

Phase 2: Knowledge Application

The second phase of the core competency is applying the knowledge developed in the first level to the practice arena. Phase two begins the APN's journey in assessing real ethical problems and being actively involved in the process of resolving ethical dilemmas. Institutional resources such as ethics committees and institutional review boards provide valuable opportunities for APNs to participate in the discussion of ethical issues. Typically, hospital ethics committees serve three functions: policy formation, case review, and education (Spencer, 1997). As the APN acquires core ethical decision-making knowledge the responsibility to take moral action becomes more compelling. Rather than retrospectively analyzing ethical dilemmas, moral action implies that the APN pursues and responds to ethical issues. Resolutions that originate from collaborative processes are more satisfactory, generate more creative solutions, and strengthen relationships (Spielman, 1993). Although the core knowledge of ethical concepts such as respect for person, truthfulness, and beneficence provide the foundation for moral reasoning, the practical application of these concepts enables the APN to evolve the practical wisdom of moral reasoning.

Phase 3: Creating an Ethical Environment

As the APN becomes more skilled in the application of ethical knowledge, the third phase of competence begins to develop. The ability to teach and mentor others regarding ethical decision making and creating an ethical environment is expected of more experienced APNs. The experienced APN may initiate informal learning opportunities for nurses and other professional colleagues. Ethics rounds and case review are two ways to engage colleagues in the discussion of moral issues. Often the roots of interdisciplinary conflict in the clinical setting are based on preconceived stereotypes of the moral viewpoints of other disciplines (Shannon, 1997). This important role of the APN also encompasses aspects of coaching, and teaching patients and families the principles of ethical decision making. It is not sufficient for the APN to simply provide information to patients and families facing difficult moral choices and expect them to arrive at a comfortable decision. The ethical competency is linked closely with the abilities to mobilize patients and move those needing help through the necessary steps to reach resolution. The APN helps others appreciate the issues and understand various ways to interpret the problem. As APNs become more competent and capable in ethical reasoning, they are able to anticipate situations in which moral conflicts occur and recognize the more subtle presentations of moral dilemmas.

Preventive Ethics. Ethical decision-making skills enable the APN to focus on identifying the values in conflict and developing a course of action suitable to the parties in dispute. An additional important role of the APN is to extend the concept of ethical decision making beyond problem-solving individual cases and move toward a paradigm of preventive ethics.

Preventive ethics is derived from the model of preventive medicine (Forrow, Arnold, & Parker, 1993). An ethical environment fosters early identification of issues and anticipation of possible dilemmas. The ability to predict areas of conflict and develop plans in a proactive, rather than reactive, manner will avert some potentially difficult dilemmas (Benner, 1991; Forrow, Arnold, & Parker, 1993). When value conflicts arise, resolution is more difficult because one value must be chosen over another. Preventive ethics emphasizes that all important values should be reviewed and examined prior to the conflict so that situations in which values may differ can be anticipated (Forrow, Arnold, & Parker, 1993).

Creating an Ethically Sensitive Environment. APNs should strive to develop environments that encourage patients and caregivers to express diverse views and raise questions about the ethical elements of clinical care. Thoughtful ethical decision making arises from an environment that supports and values the critical exchange of ideas and promotes collaboration among members of the health care team, patients, and families. A collaborative practice environment in turn supports shared decision making, shared accountability, and group participation, and it fosters relationships based on equality and mutuality (Pike, 1991). The APN is integral in the development and preservation of a collaborative climate that inspires and empowers individuals to respond to moral dilemmas. The APN should advocate for a process of ongoing, rather than episodic, ethical inquiry. This approach to moral reflection sanctions open discussions of values and divergent views and is realized through the reciprocal exchanges of information between members of the health care team and the patient.

Acquiring and Developing Ethical Decision-Making Competencies

The skills needed to identify, articulate, and address ethical dilemmas are complex and diverse. Particular strategies, such as those used in values clarification, negotiation, and mediation, provide a foundation for the practice aspects of ethical decision making. The APN must understand the theoretical elements of biomedical ethics and be aware of paradigm cases and relevant law to interpret moral issues in the health care setting. However, successful resolution of moral issues will more likely occur if the application of ethical knowledge is tempered with compassionate and effective communication skills.

Overview of Ethical Theories

Although ethical decision making in health care is extensively discussed in the bioethics literature, two dominant models most often are applied in the clinical setting. The analytical model of decision making is a principle-based model. In this model, ethical decision making is guided by theories, principles, and rules (Beauchamp & Childress, 1994). In cases of conflict, the principles or rules in contention are balanced and interpreted with the contextual elements of the circumstance. However, the final decision and moral justification for actions are based on an appeal to principles. In this way, the principles are both binding and tolerant of the particularities of specific cases (Beauchamp & Childress, 1994; Childress, 1994).

The principles of respect for persons, autonomy, beneficence, nonmaleficence, and justice are commonly applied in the analysis of ethical issues in nursing. The ANA's current *Code for Nurses* (2001) embraces the principle of respect for persons and underscores the profession's commitment to service. The emphasis on respect for persons throughout the *Code* implies that it is not only a philosophical value of nursing but also a binding principle within the profession. Although ethical principles and rules are the cornerstone of most ethical decisions, the principle-based approach has been criticized as too formalistic and rigorous for many clinicians (Ahronheim, Moreno, & Zuckerman, 1994).

PRINCIPLES AND RULES IMPORTANT TO PROFESSIONAL NURSING PRACTICE	
Principle of Respect for Autonomy	The duty to respect others' personal liberty and individual values, beliefs, and choices
Principle of Nonmaleficence	The duty not to inflict harm or evil
Principle of Beneficence	The duty to do good and prevent or remove harm
Principle of Formal Justice	The duty to treat equals equally and treat those who are unequal according to their needs
Rule of Veracity	The duty to tell the truth and not to deceive others
Rule of Fidelity	The duty to honor commitments
Rule of Confidentiality	The duty not to disclose information shared in an intimate and trusted manner
Rule of Privacy	The duty to respect limited access to a person

Definitions adapted from Beauchamp, T.L., Childress, J.F. (1994). *Principles of biomedical ethics* (4th ed.) New York: Oxford University Press.

Critics argue that a principle-based approach conceals the particular person and relationships and reduces the resolution of a clinical case to simply balancing principles (Gudorf, 1994). Consequently, when conflicts among principles occur, the description of the principle is inadequate to provide guidance for resolving the dilemma (Ahronheim, Moreno, & Zuckerman, 1994; Childress, 1994).

A second approach to ethical decision making is the casuistic model, in which current cases are compared with paradigm cases (Aronheim, Moreno, & Zuckerman, 1994; Beauchamp & Childress, 1994; Jonsen & Toulmin, 1988; Toulmin, 1994). The strength of this approach is that dilemmas are examined in a context-specific manner and then compared with an analogous earlier case. The fundamental philosophical assumption of this model is that ethics emerges from human moral experiences (Ahronheim et al., 1994;

Jonsen & Toulmin, 1988). The casuists approach dilemmas from an inductive position and work from the specific case to generalizations, rather than from generalizations to specific cases (Ahronheim et al., 1994; Beauchamp & Childress, 1994; Gaul, 1995).

Some concerns arise when evaluating a casuistic model for ethical decision making. As a moral dilemma arises, the selection of the paradigm case may differ among the decision makers, and thus the interpretation of the appropriate course of action will vary. Furthermore, other than the reliance on previous cases, casuists have no mechanisms to justify their actions. The possibility that previous cases were reasoned in a faulty or inaccurate manner is not considered or evaluated (Beauchamp & Childress, 1994).

Other theories, such as utilitarianism, Kantianism, virtue-based theory, and care-based theory provide alternative processes for moral reflection and argument (Beauchamp & Childress, 1994). In particular, the ethics of care has emerged as relevant to nursing (Cooper, 1989). The care perspective constructs moral problems as issues surrounding the intrinsic needs and corresponding responsibilities that occur within relationships (Cooper, 1989; Gilligan, 1982). Moral reasoning involves empathy and emphasizes responsibility rather than rights. The response of the individual to a moral dilemma emerges from the affiliate relationship and the norms of friendship, care, and love (Beauchamp & Childress, 1994; Cooper, 1989). Although every ethical theory has some limitations and problems, an understanding of contemporary approaches to ethics and bioethics is a central feature in achieving a moral resolution. Moral reasoning most often reflects a blend of the various theories rather than the application of a single theory.

Ethical Decision Making

Acquiring the skills and competence to facilitate the resolution of moral dilemmas is an evolutionary process. Because ethical decision making is not exclusively based on theoretical knowledge, moral reasoning must be tempered with clinical reality. As APNs gain the necessary knowledge and skills in ethical decision making, their involvement should intensify and become more extensive. One procedural framework nurses can use in ethical decision making is to adapt the nursing process as a framework to organize and guide the gathering of morally relevant information. This enables the APN to systematically organize the facts and contextual particularities of a dilemma. Although a framework provides structure and suggests a method of examining and studying the ethical issues, the essential component to resolution of ethical dilemmas is moral action. Simply knowing the right course of action does not guarantee that a person has the motivation or courage to act (Rest, 1986). Successful resolution of moral issues requires a blend of knowledge, conviction, emotions, beliefs, and individual character (van Hooft, 1990).

Problem Identification

Ethical dilemmas often are first recognized by the intense emotional reactions they elicit. A difficult but important step in problem identification is to allow and encourage the individuals in conflict to openly express their emotions. This action demonstrates that the perspectives and the emotional responses to the issue are legitimate and meaningful (Fisher & Ury, 1981). As a facilitator, the APN should recognize, understand, and acknowledge the emotions of all parties.

Many conflicts that arise in the clinical setting generate powerful emotional responses yet may not be ethical issues. Ethical issues involve some form of controversy concerning moral values (Ahronheim, Moreno, & Zuckerman, 1994). It is essential that the APN distinguish and separate moral dilemmas from other issue such as administrative concerns, communication problems, or lack of clinical knowledge. Identifying the cause of the problem and determining why, where, and when it occurred, as well as who or what was affected, will help clarify the nature of the problem (Beare, 1989).

Information Gathering

Once the ethical problem is identified, the APN implements a process to gather and examine the morally relevant facts. Generally, information such as the medical and nursing facts; the values, rights, and obligations of the patient; legal factors; and cultural and religious factors should be gathered when initiating the decision-making process. However, these facts are insufficient if not tempered with the contextual features of each case. Only after the unique conditions of the case are considered can an ethically acceptable solution be identified.

Strategies for Resolution

Moral discussions and deliberation can take the form of a debate that degenerates into an assault. One party presents an argument, the other party disputes it, the original party defends, and the second party attacks (Zaner, 1988). Breaking this cycle of destructive interactions is central to arriving at solutions that are resourceful and constructive. Resolutions are most effective when the parties in dispute create the solution.

When the APN is directly involved in a conflict situation, the skills of negotiation are most useful in moving toward a satisfactory settlement. However, in cases where resolution is not easily achieved, it is best to solicit help from a member of the ethics committee or another professional colleague not involved in the case.

The challenge in most cases of ethical disputes is to have all involved listen to each other's perspectives in order to understand the basis of the disagreement and to work together to create a collaborative solution (Saulo & Wagener, 1996). In many cases, the APN must serve as a facilitator for the parties in dispute and apply the strategies involved in mediation. The key difference between these roles is the level of active involvement in deciding the goals and strategies of resolving the dilemma. As a negotiating party, the APN suggests solutions and identifies acceptable plans (Beare, 1989). In the role of a mediator, the APN guides the process but does not offer opinions or solutions (Ostermeyer, 1991). The process and steps used in negotiation and mediation overlap in many ways, and in both approaches the parties in conflict discover and determine the acceptable solutions (Beare, 1989; Ostermeyer, 1991).

The objective of successful negotiation and mediation is to achieve a mutually satisfactory solution. In reality, however, that is not always possible. The issues of time, cost, available resources, level of moral certainty and the perceived value of the relationship play important roles in the strategy used and likelihood of reaching a desired outcome (Spielman, 1993). The key role of the APN in the resolution of moral dilemmas is to guide and stimulate communication between the differing parties. The following strategies for negotiation are useful when the APN is facilitating resolution between two parties and when the professional or personal values of the APN collide with the values of others.

Collaboration

Collaboration is the preferred strategy for achieving a moral resolution. The first step in the process of collaboration is to help the disputing parties agree on the issue in conflict and to understand both the cognitive and the emotional perspectives of each party. Because emotions maintain a significant position in moral dilemmas, it is important to provide an environment in which the parties can release unexpressed emotions. An effective method to help others resolve anger or frustration is to listen in a nonjudgmental manner and avoid reacting to the criticism (Fisher & Ury, 1981). Discussions that occur after the release of emotions are more rational and productive because the emotions have been expressed in an explicit and unambiguous manner (Fisher & Ury, 1981). The APN encourages the parties to discuss their perception of the problem, recognize their emotions, and identify their expectations for resolution (Krouse & Roberts, 1989).

The second step toward successful collaborative moral resolution is to engage all involved parties in active interactions and consensus building (Krouse & Roberts, 1989). Information presented should be questioned, analyzed, and examined. It is important to focus on the interests of each party rather than the positions. Asking the questions "why?" and "why not?" can identify interests of the involved individuals (Fisher & Ury, 1981). As differing interests emerge, the varying perspectives should be acknowledged with confidence and hopefulness (Ury, 1993). The parties must listen to each other but need not necessarily agree on the others' views or on what is being said. From this stage of active communication and interaction, the process of consensus building begins.

The third step in negotiating or mediating a moral resolution involves formulating a decision and developing a plan. The objective of both negotiation and mediation is to generate options and solutions that are consistent with all parties' principles and achieve an outcome that is mutually satisfying (Ostermeyer, 1991; Ury, 1993). During this phase, the parties explore options and together decide on a plan of action. Initially this joint negotiation may seem unlikely, particularly when both parties are attached to their own positions. However, it is possible for the APN to facilitate progression through complex situations by using communication skills such as reframing, identifying shared interests and needs, and examining the differences (Fisher & Ury, 1981; Smeltzer, 1991).

Compromise

When both parties possess a high level of moral certainty in their positions and are committed to preserving the relationship, they may choose to bargain each relinquish some control over the decision. Compromising and bargaining are time consuming because each party must determine what are acceptable trade-offs. Because time in the clinical setting is limited, both parties must value the relationship and share in the decision making process (Spielman, 1993).

Problems are resolved through compromise when both parties are willing to waive some components of their moral position and embrace a position of cooperation (Spielman, 1993). For example, a chronically ill patient with dilated cardiomyopathy may refuse in-hospital management of the heart failure but agree to a short-term solution, such as a trial of intravenous therapy at home.

Accomodation

In some cases, one party will accommodate and simply agree to support the other's position. This approach may indicate that, to one party, the issue in question was too insignificant for her or him to strive for a mutually acceptable solution (Spielman, 1993). Accommodation frequently occurs when the issue is trivial, time is limited, or one party holds a high level of commitment to preserving the relationship with the other participant (Spielman, 1993). Accommodation is sometimes employed as a tactic in negotiation. The concession is made to dissipate friction and additionally to imply that a reciprocal action is expected in future negotiations with the other party. However, accommodation is an inappropriate strategy when used routinely to gain acceptance or merely to avoid conflict.

Coercion

A coercive and controlling approach may be used when time is short, such as in an emergency, or when the party has little commitment to the relationship. This approach is often aggressive and competitive and reflects a high degree of commitment to a particular moral position (Spielman, 1993). Because control of the decision is assumed by one party and the differing perspectives are discounted, this approach damages the self-esteem of the other party and may result in a sense of powerlessness and moral outrage (Pike, 1991).

An environment in which a coercive and controlling approach is prevalent generates a power imbalance that accentuates vulnerability. Vulnerability damages self-esteem, constrains independence, and restricts choices (Copp, 1986). In this environment, relationships have little importance, and it is unlikely that the group with authority will actively pursue empowering the vulnerable group. Change can occur in this climate, but it often emanates from the constrained party. Redefining one's position (i.e., from victim to involved decision maker) and acknowledging accountability and responsibility for reaching collaborative resolutions are strategies to alter a coercive environment (Pike, 1991).

Avoidance

Participants may avoid, ignore, or deny the dilemma when the moral issue is perceived as trivial or, conversely, is deeply felt by one party and highly charged emotionally. Avoidance is also seen when time is short (Spielman, 1993). If a decision is unnecessary, it may be appropriate for a participant to withdraw from the process of decision making. However, this strategy often is employed when the participant abdicates moral accountability. The APN should consciously monitor avoidance behaviors and pursue the rationale for this technique. It is likely that the individuals who practice this technique regularly avoid conflict and would benefit from additional knowledge, support, and role modeling of approaches to conflict management. Individuals who consistently evade moral dilemmas may benefit from values clarification exercises to help them explore deeply held values and to learn ways to deal with them more productively.

Evaluation of Ethical Decision Making

The evaluation of ethical decision making should focus on two areas: the process and the outcome. Process evaluation is important because it provides an overview of the moral disagreement, the interpersonal skills employed, the interactions between both parties in conflict, and the problems encountered during the phases of resolution. Evaluation of the outcome is also critical because it acknowledges creative solutions and celebrates moral action. Other components of the outcome evaluation include the short-term and long-term consequences of the action taken and the satisfaction of all parties with the chosen solution (Olczak, Grosch, & Duffy, 1991). Unfortunately, a successful process does not always result in a satisfactory outcome. Occasionally the outcomes reveal the need for changes within the institution or health care system. The goal of the outcome evaluation is to minimize the risks of a similar event by identifying predictable patterns and thereby averting recurrent and future dilemmas.

The APN is in a key position to assume a more decisive role in managing the resolution of moral issues. The skills of problem identification, values clarification, negotiation, collaboration, and evaluation empower the APN to critically analyze and direct the decision making process. The identification of patterns in the presentation of moral issues will enable the APN to engage in preventive strategies to improve the ethical qualities of patient care.

The Clinical Nurse Specialist in Action 4

The Clinical Nurse Specialist

The Clinical Nurse Specialist (CNS) is a registered nurse "who, through study and supervised practice at the graduate level (master's or doctorate), has become expert in a defined area of knowledge and practice in a selected clinical area of nursing" (American Nurses Association, 1980, p. 23). The dimensions of the CNS role are expert clinician, consultant, educator, and researcher. The CNS role was created to keep expert nurses in clinical practice and to improve patient care. The intent of the CNS role is to improve patient care and influence others. CNSs are successful when they deliver high-quality care that can be measured in terms of cost-effectiveness, patient outcomes, and improvements in nursing practice. In 1989, Hamric proposed the CNS role definition, using a three-dimensional model to delineate the role's defining characteristics and the relationships between primary criteria for the role (e.g., graduate study in the specialty, certification, and focus of practice on the patient/client/family), the four subroles (clinical expert, consultant, educator, and researcher), and skills or competencies (e.g., change agent, collaborator, clinical leader, role model, patient advocate) (Hamric, 1989a).

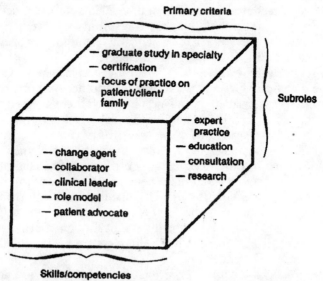

Figure 1-1. Defining characteristics of the CNS role.

From Hamric, A.B. (1989). History and overview of the CNS role, *The Clinical Nurse Specialist in Theory and Practice*. Philadelphia:? W.B Saunders Company, p. 8.

CNS Competencies and Spheres of Influence

The classic dimensions or subroles of the CNS are expert clinician, consultant, change agent (leader), educator, and researcher. Integrating these dimensions is difficult but necessary, yet maintaining distinction between the elements is important to keep role responsibilities clear (Sparacino & Cooper, 1990). There are competencies, or skills, that a CNS must master to accomplish and integrate the subroles. Some competencies are common threads that weave throughout core competencies, such as clinical and professional leadership, collaboration, and ethical decision making. The core competencies include direct and indirect clinical practice, consulting, expert teaching and coaching, and scholarly or scientific inquiry. What the CNS does (i.e., the four subroles) and how the CNS performs the role (i.e., competencies) can have a substantial impact on the practice setting (i.e., spheres of influence). Practice in each sphere of influence (patients/clients, nurses, and organizations/networks) (NACNS, 1998), in combination with mastery of CNS competencies, is essential to be a successful CNS.

CNS Competencies

Clinical Practice. Clinical practice is the heart of advanced nursing practice. A CNS is most likely to directly care for a patient whose diagnosis or care is complex, unique, or problematic. A CNS's clinical expertise and specialty influence the patient population to whom care is given. Direct clinical practice is also a means by which the CNS can assess the quality of care for a specific patient population; it provides a qualitative assessment that enhances the interpretation of quantitative data and directs the change in care provided. The type of care a CNS gives is either regular or episodic (Koetters, 1989). Involvement in regular or episodic care enables the CNS to identify problems that interfere with care and require CNS intervention. Examples include lack of staff knowledge, need for clinical policies or procedures, or the need for conflict mediation among team members. For each clinical situation, a CNS takes a comprehensive approach and uses a high level of discriminative judgment, advanced knowledge, and expert skill, including expertise in the technical and humanistic aspects of care. Although clinical expertise is the cornerstone of CNS practice, a CNS will not be successful because of knowledge or technical expertise alone. A CNS's clinical practice interventions may be continuous or time limited, but should result in improvements in clinical outcomes, patient/family satisfaction, resource allocation, staff knowledge and skills, health care team collaboration, and organizational efficiency.

A CNS also regularly provides indirect care, for example, when a CNS delegates care to but guides the direct care given by a staff nurse. Another type of indirect patient care occurs when a CNS selects a patient population in which there are recurrent problems or themes, poor outcomes, or recidivism, and then collaborates with other members of the health care team to develop and implement standards of care, critical pathways, clinical procedures, or quality or performance improvement plans. Implementation and adherence should be evaluated in order to compare outcomes; refine clinical pathways, algorithms, or guidelines; improve clinical management; and further promote consistent adherence. A pathway or guidelines is rarely self-sustaining, and requires a key person who continuously champions implementation if it is to be successful and achieve its intended outcomes. A CNS is often the primary coordinator of such an effort. Another type of indirect patient care provided by the CNS is related to system responsibilities for evaluating technology and its impact on patients and resources.

Consulting. The CNS is a content expert and so assists in suggesting a wide range of alternative approaches or solutions to clinical or systems problems, whether internal or external to the practice setting. The CNS is a resource consultant who provides pertinent information that enables nurses and others to make decisions based on a range of relevant and appropriate alternatives. The CNS is a process consultant who facilitates change so that decisions can be made for particular and future situations (Sparacino & Cooper, 1990). A CNS can be an internal and external consultant. Internal consultation is part of the CNS job description and includes assisting with organizational development in one's own practice setting, especially the creative use of resources and alternative strategies to bypass perceived system obstacles. A CNS may recognize that an internal consultation needs the collaboration of multiple consultants, with more than one CNS and other disciplines participating; a CNS often initiates the plan, mobilizes the resources, defuses the politics, and facilitates the resolution. Unless consultation is a CNS's primary responsibility, there may be a problem if a CNS's time is used more for consultations than direct care and the impact on patient care is less visible, unless the strategies are well documented and the outcomes measured.

External consultation assists the nursing profession, a specialty organization, other health providers, and health systems external to the practice setting with approaches or solutions for specific problems. The consultant aspect of the CNS role is not necessarily a given; it is an expectation, but each CNS's consultative skill varies. Consultation requires interpersonal skills of flexibility, trust, and a nonjudgmental and nonthreatening demeanor. The goal of consultation is to help the consultee become more knowledgeable.

Expert Teaching and Coaching. Expert teaching and coaching is a part of direct clinical practice and is influenced by scholarly inquiry and research utilization. The CNS teaching and coaching function is both formal and informal. A CNS teaches staff nurses, patients and families, graduate nursing students, clinical nurse specialists, health professionals, and consumer groups. Expert coaching implies "the existence of a relationship that is fundamental to effective teaching" (Clarke & Spross, 1996, p. 140). A CNS is a role model for nurses, demonstrating the practical integration of theory and evidence-based practice. By maintaining a focus on continuously improving clinical practice and integrating new knowledge into practice, a CNS influences the further development of the proficient, expert nurse, and increases the staff nurse's accountability and autonomy. A staff nurse can become the role model for the skill mastered or the knowledge gained, and so the influence of the CNS continues to improve patient care. This growth cycle is never complete. A CNS's expert teaching and coaching skills are pivotal in providing or influencing patient and family education. Teaching or coaching complements the care given to a patient and family by other nurses and health professionals. CNSs continually look for better ways to teach patients and families, using diverse combinations of cognitive, educational, and behavioral strategies to improve patient education and compliance. However, a CNS may not be able to teach every patient and family and so must assess whom to teach. A CNS could delegate routine teaching to a staff nurse or practice case manager, and allocate more time to teaching high-risk or complex patients. A CNS also has many opportunities to educate other health care providers and consumer groups.

Scholarly or Scientific Inquiry. The essential components of the researcher role (McGuire & Harwood, 1989; Sparacino & Cooper, 1990) and advanced practice research competencies (McGuire & Harwood, 1996) are described in the literature. The competency of scholarly or scientific inquiry encompasses the continuum from scholarly inquiry to research utilization and research conduct. A CNS fosters the spirit of inquiry by documenting problems to determine research needs or by generating or refining research problems. Inherent to the CNS role is the responsibility to interpret and apply research findings. A CNS analyzes and evaluates the appropriateness of the research, and applies research findings to clinical practice. Evidence-based practice is realized in clinical procedures, administrative policies, educational materials for patients and staff, and clinical pathways. Evaluating outcomes of practice is another important example of research application (McGuire & Harwood, 1996).

In order to be effective, CNSs must be able to apply research to practice. Research is essential to build and extend the knowledge base for nursing practice, and to better understand the impact of nursing interventions on patient outcomes. Most often the practical level of involvement is collaborative nursing and interdisciplinary research (McGuire & Harwood, 1996). By being a member of a research team, a CNS is in the unique position to contribute to the generation of clinically based knowledge, to create a link between practical application and theoretical design, and to bridge the gap between how nursing ought to be and what is current practice. A CNS is the clinical expert, understands the clinical issues, and has access to patients; a nurse researcher is the research expert, knows research methodology, and has access to the resources that support the research. CNSs and nurse researchers should actively be involved in research that documents the impact of advanced nursing practice, managed care, and other health care changes on the quality of patient care.

Clinical and Professional Leadership. The leadership competency is another of the common threads that weave throughout the core competencies. A CNS has significant formal and informal impact and influence; a CNS must be visionary yet practical. A CNS is a change agent. Through the CNS's influence and authority, nursing practice improves (Hamric, 1983b). As change agent, a CNS is the link between a variety of resources and nursing staff (Girouard, 1983), and asserts clinical and professional leadership in the practice setting or health care system, in health care policy and delivery decisions, or in the administration of direct care programs. A CNS authors and actuates clinical procedures, practice guidelines, and clinical pathways; designs and directs quality and performance improvement initiatives; chairs interdisciplinary committees or manages clinical projects; and influences or guides institutional health care policy decisions. A CNS can serve as an advocate or "shuttle diplomat" between administrators and clinical staff, helping both groups understand the vagaries and particulars of organizational change, listening and supporting when appropriate and explaining decisions when needed (Brown, 1989).

Collaboration. Collaboration is the second common thread, and it is an essential competency. A CNS collaborates with nurses, physicians, other health care providers and patients and their families. A CNS is a nurse attending, a teacher and role model for nursing staff. The outcome of CNS-coordinated collaboration is empowerment of nurses and a recognition of the nurse as a critical member of the health care team (Boyle, 1996). This results in team building, synergism, and integrative solutions. CNSs and physicians also collaborate, although some practice settings and working relationships are more enlightened or conducive to partnership than others. When boundary issues and the pragmatic considerations of jobs and income are put aside, the differences in physician and CNS practice are complementary, afford integrative solutions, and further strengthen collaboration (Minarik & Sparacino, 1990). The outcome is high-quality and cost-efficient care. A CNS builds collaborative relationships with patients and families and provides an interface between patient, family, and physician. A CNS is in the unique position to assist a patient and family to determine their needs, assess treatment options, and ensure a positive outcome. CNS advocacy often prevents adversarial situations and their negative sequelae.

Ethical Decision Making. Ethical decision making is a specific APN competency; it is also a common thread running through all core competencies. A CNS has significant influence on the negotiation of moral dilemma, direction of patient care, access to care, and allocation of resources. CNSs consider numerous factors when making ethical decisions, including professional and religious codes, cultural values, bioethical principles, the casuistic model, and ethical theories (Reigle, 1996). CNSs play critical roles in preventive and applied ethics. In promoting preventive ethics, a CNS is responsible for anticipating ethical conflicts when possible, teaching ethical theories, helping staff and patients clarify values, serving as a role model in discussions with patients about treatment preferences and options, demonstrating critical thinking in the analysis of moral dilemmas, and enhancing others' autonomy (Forrow, Arnold, & Parker, 1993, cited in Reigle, 1996).

CNSs have similar responsibilities when applying ethical decision-making skills to patient and organizational issues. They can articulate moral dilemmas. They can interpret and mediate patient, family, and team members' perspectives to ensure as complete a discussion as possible. They recognize the need for consultation with an ethics committee and often initiate the consult. When necessary, CNSs validate staff nurses' concerns and help nurses present their concerns to other team members, ensuring that the nursing perspective is considered when ethical issues are discussed. When CNSs are excluded from interdisciplinary processes involving ethical decisions, opportunities for effective nursing care are minimized and outcomes such as timely and appropriate end-of-life care are compromised (Oddi & Cassidy, 1998).

Spheres of Influence

Having described CNS competencies, it is apparent that there are three spheres of CNS influence: patient/clients, nursing personnel, and organizations or networks (NACNS, 1998). CNSs influence the patient/client sphere through activities such as assessment; diagnosis, planning, and outcome identification; interventions; and evaluation. CNSs influence nursing personnel by helping to identify and define problems and opportunities in delivering care, nurse-specific outcomes, and collaborative practice; developing innovative solutions; and evaluating the effect of those solutions. The organization/network sphere of influence includes identifying problems and opportunities, identifying resource management needs and developing innovative solutions, and evaluating the quality and cost-effectiveness of patient care technologies and care processes (NACNS, 1998).

The delineation of spheres of influence is theoretically intended to avoid the overlap of subrole competencies and the perception of role ambiguity by distinguishing CNSs from other APNs (NACNS, 1998). Each sphere of influence requires various CNS competencies, so what a CNS does (i.e., the four subroles) and how a CNS performs the role (i.e. competencies) affects the practice setting through the effective use of influence (i.e., spheres of influence). Understanding each sphere of influence and mastering CNS competencies are essential for a CNS to be successful.

Impact and Influence

A CNS plays a significant role in any health care delivery system by keeping a comprehensive focus on quality care and extensive documentation to facilitate quality patient outcomes. Managed care has provided CNSs with an opportunity that has long eluded them: linking their services to patient outcomes and resource utilization. A CNS's particular impact has been on patient and family outcomes, outcomes management, care efficiency, and cost-effectiveness. However, prevention of patient care variance is difficult to quantify.

Evidence-Based Practice

Knowledge is the basis for practice. When research is evaluated for its applicable scientific evidence, informed decisions are made in providing patient care and achieving good patient outcomes, and credible nursing practice is documented (McPheeters & Lohr, 1999). A CNS is the ideal clinician to assess the contextual factors that are barriers and facilitators to change, and to develop and implement evidence-based practice. In addition, a CNS's involvement in the development of clinical pathways and procedures means that the CNS can ensure research evidence informs clinical processes and standards.

Outcomes Management

Management of outcomes is driven by the rapid movement to managed care, and the need for national standards for measuring performance in health care. Traditionally, key outcome indicators have been linked more to organizational structures than to organizational or clinical processes. Although key outcome indicators are influenced by patient variables more than organizational variables, less attention has been given to the relationship between organizational attributes and patient outcomes (Mitchell & Shortell, 1997). The traditional model linking structure, processes, and outcome is a linear one, but Mitchell, Ferketich, and Jennings (1998) proposed a dynamic model that posits reciprocal relationships between the care delivery system, interventions, clients, and outcomes. Assuming responsibility for using outcome data to improve patient care delivery is a prime opportunity for the CNS to assess patient care strategies and community systems, analyze interdisciplinary communication and collaboration, coordinate care, monitor patient and system progress, and evaluate patient and system outcomes. The challenge is to facilitate cost-effective patient care interventions that are effective with all populations.

CNS Impact on Outcomes

Measuring and reporting the impact of a CNS on patient and family outcomes has been slow, but the evidence is mounting and the impact irrefutable. Classic studies include evaluation of the impact of CNS interventions on low-birth-weight infants (Brooten et al., 1986) and hospitalized elderly patients (Neidlinger, Kennedy, & Scroggins, 1987). More recent studies have demonstrated the impact of CNS interventions on patients who received transitional care services from a CNS and were discharged from the hospital earlier than the norm; the impact of CNS practice specifically related to case management or outcomes management demonstrate cost savings, patient satisfaction, and increased staff knowledge.

Issues and Challenges

A number of issues currently challenge the CNS role. These issues include but are not limited to educational preparation; factors influencing role evolution, such as health care organizational changes and forced changes in role focus and titling; second licensure; and legal barriers.

Educational Preparation

The dilemma in defining appropriate CNS education has been the identification of and agreement about a core body of knowledge for practice. All agree that basic CNS preparation requires a master's degree in nursing.

Factors Influencing CNS Role Evolution

Organizational Considerations. A classic but recurring debate is whether a CNS should be in a staff or a line position (Prouty, 1983; Baird & Prouty, 1989). In a staff position, a CNS is freed from more administrative responsibilities and allowed to focus on patient care delivery and related issues, and the less threatening consultative capacity. The disadvantage of such a position is a lack of formal authority, such that power is referent or exercised by virtue of clinical expertise and knowledge. The advantage for a CNS in a line position is formal authority, but the distinct disadvantage is that administrative responsibilities may dominate one's activities and erode the time available for clinical issues and patient care.

Recently there has been serious discussion about the need for a CNS to acquire NP skills for job security. The basis for this challenge may be that CNSs have been increasingly pulled from the bedside to address competing demands and other organizational needs. Those who disagree with this proposal argue that an acute care NP's (ACNP) primary emphasis is on patient care, limited to the particular practice setting and to the exclusion of a CNS's flexibility to care for patients across the continuum of care. In addition, the ACNP has less opportunity to participate in other areas of usual CNS influence, such as staff education and development, nurse mentorship, change agent leadership, consultation, research, and outcomes management.

The CNS as Case Manager. The minimum educational requirement endorsed by the Case Management Society of America for a nurse case manager is a baccalaureate degree. However, a master's prepared case manager who also has experience as a CNS is very effective because case management includes many CNS responsibilities, such as patient care, collaboration with a multidisciplinary team, clinical system orchestration, administration of the interface between a patient and the health care system, and involvement with, if not direction of, resource management and clinical system development. However, managed care's impact affects resource management and CNS impact and influence, especially if a CNS is used exclusively as a case manager. In such situations, the APN case manager is forced to neglect CNS responsibilities such as coaching of nurses.

The CNS as Outcomes Manager. There is a theoretical but subtle distinction between a case manager and an outcomes manager. A case manager's responsibilities are unit or setting-based and involve coordinating patient-focused care and resource management. An outcomes manager's responsibilities are broader, including additional obligations that focus on the continuum of care that is beyond a specific case load. An outcomes manager is responsible for clinical and financial analysis and outcomes for a particular patient population, including development and revision of organizational systems. The literature suggests that a CNS, with her or his expert clinical and consultant competencies, is best qualified to be an outcomes manager and to undertake the responsibilities of patient and quality measurement and research, financial analysis, provider education, and development and implementation of interdisciplinary practice improvements (Houston & Luquire, 1997; Weiss, 1998).

Second Licensure

An alternative to second licensure is a multistate licensure system proposed by the National Council of State Boards of Nursing (NCSBN) in 1997 (NCSBN, 1998). An interstate compact addresses the more general licensure issues that hinder interstate practice, making mobility between two or more states possible while keeping a state-based licensure and discipline agreement. The interstate compact has not yet addressed advanced practice, in part because there is little licensure uniformity for advanced practice (Williamson & Hutcherson, 1998).

Legal Barriers

Legal barriers for a CNS are similar to those encountered by other advanced practice nurses: restrictions on scope of practice, authority to prescribe drugs, and reimbursement. Although Safriet's classic monograph addressed NP and certified nurse-midwife issues, her recommendations are also applicable to a CNS's expanding domain and scope of practice. However, CNSs must consider how general or specific desired regulatory changes should be. Although progress has been made in overcoming the barriers imposed by state statutes and administrative dicta, the financial changes in the current health care market have created new challenges for APNs in general, and CNSs in particular (Safriet, 1998).

Evaluating the Role

Evaluating CNS effectiveness in a way that links structural and process variables is useful only if the procedure also addresses CNS impact on cost, quality, and patient outcomes (Girouard, 1996). Common elements include CNS impact on patient care quality and cost of patient outcomes, with similar results regardless of specialty area or practice setting (Barnason et al, 1998; Broussard, 1996; Mathew et al., 1994; McAlpine, 1997).

The CNS Case Manager

Driven largely by economics, the goal of managed care is to deliver cost-effective care through prudent use of resources and the elimination of redundant and unnecessary services. A variety of medical management techniques to improve care and contain costs in the competitive health care market have been implemented. These include utilization management, critical pathways, patient care guidelines, and case management.

Not only will APN case managers perform the traditional case management activities of assessing, planning, implementing, and coordinating activities for individuals with immediate health care needs, they also will find themselves engaged in population-based programs for high-risk client groups who have no active symptoms or complications. Nurse case managers (NCMs) will be educating, supporting, coaching, and advocating for clients at risk for chronic disease and other high-risk health problems so that those clients adopt behaviors known to reduce disease, limit chronicity or progression, and prevent complications. Not only willAPN case managers be challenged to demonstrate cost savings, they also will be called upon to use empirical techniques to show that the case management process does indeed influence client behaviors, clinical outcomes, and physical and emotional functioning.

Case Management

Case management is a practice framework that has been implemented in a variety of settings by nurses, social workers, and other health care providers. To foster a common understanding of the work done by professional case managers, the interdisciplinary Case Management Society of America (CMSA) has defined case management as "A collaborative process which assesses, plans, implements, coordinates, monitors and evaluates options and services to meet an individual's health needs through communications and available resources to promote quality cost-effective outcomes" (CMSA, 1994, p.8). This definition incorporates the system, clinical, and fiscal aspects that are central to case management approaches to providing care.

APN Case Management

Contemporary nurse case management reflects a natural evolution from nursing's history of client advocacy, social service, and public health. APNs also provide care that is congruent with case management concepts; their care can improve health care access, coordination, and continuity across settings (Brooten et al., 1991; Newman, 1990; Office of Technology Assessment, 1986). Such studies suggest that APN case management is a means of improving access to care in a timely manner. APN case management also has been viewed as a way of enhancing the visibility of advanced nursing practice (Cooper, 1990; Hamric, 1992; Mahn & Spross, 1996). Many arguments have been made for assigning nurse case management to APNs (Connors, 1993; Fralic, 1992; Hamric, 1992). Currently the APN CM is an evolving advanced practice role, and has yet to be formally recognized by the ANA as advanced nursing practice. The APN CM is master's prepared and must have expert knowledge in a clinical specialty, the skills to establish mutually agreeable goals between the client and other members of the health care team, and the ability to establish an intervention schema that will help the client reach his or her goals. However, the scope of influence of the APN CM differs from other APN roles, in that the APN CM is expected to influence care at a systems level through establishing disease management strategies, health promotion, disease prevention, and complication management programs across the continuum of health care services. Finally, the APN CM is accountable for evaluating the effectiveness of the case management intervention, both at the level of an individual patient/client and at a system-wide level.

Managed Care Trends

Care Reimbursement Trends. Managed care is an integrated network that combines the financing and delivery of health care services to covered individuals. Conceptually, there is a triad of players associated with any managed care organization – the payer, the hospital providers, and the physician providers. Generally, the managed care organization serves as the payer, and contracts with health care organizations and physicians to furnish health care services to members of the plan. In managed care, financial incentives exist that encourage members to use providers associated with the plan and to follow procedures that help the plan to control costs. Financial incentives also encourage providers to control expenditures.

The NCM must be able to recognize the discrepancies among multiple reimbursement structures that affect decision making for the clients for whom she or he is responsible. To complicate the matter even further, the NCM must also be aware that financial incentives among hospitals, providers, and payers are often far from aligned. For example, an agreement may exist between a hospital and a payer to provide services under a capitated agreement. However, if the patient's physician is reimbursed under a traditional fee-for-service structure, it may be difficult to motivate the physician to reduce admissions or LOS. In addition, there may be few economic incentives for the physician to limit use of medically prescribed resources, which account for most health care expenses. NCMs may then find themselves in a situation of conflict between the medical providers and the health care organization. Likewise, NCMs may find themselves in a situation of conflict between the needs of the patients and the payer. In these situations, NCMs need to be able to influence decisions made by other stakeholders through their expertise in clinical assessment and articulation of the patient's needs in order to secure the most appropriate health care settings and services.

Regulatory Requirements. The constraints of a cost-managed system are becoming increasingly problematic. Managed care systems are expected to have explicit standards for selection of their care providers and formal programs for quality improvement and utilization review. Increasingly, regulatory requirements are being applied to managed care organizations, who not only have to prove a profit margin to their stockholders, but must be able to demonstrate quality of care to employers and other purchases of health care.

Risk-Assessing a Population for Targeted Case Management Interventions. A small percentage of individuals often account for the disproportionate share of health care expenditures. In a typical population, 5% of the members (most of whom are severely, chronically ill) consume 6% of the health care costs, 45% of the members consume 37% of the costs, and the remaining 50% of the population account for only 3% of the costs (unpublished data from Value Health Sciences, Inc., Santa Monica, CA, June 1995, cited in Eichert, Wong, and Smith, 1997, p. 41). A closer review of these resource-intense populations reveals three subgroups of patient/member types. First, there are those patients who have had a single high-expense episode, such as organ transplant, total joint replacement, or heart valve surgery. A second group is comprised of patients with terminal disease who are resource intensive for a finite period of time. The third group is comprised of patients with chronic disease, such as diabetes, renal failure, hypertension, or asthma, who ultimately utilize a large portion of health care goods and services (C.J. Heller, personal communication, 1999).

Within the chronic disease group, there are three further subcategories of individuals. The first subcategory is those patients/members who are medically unstable and who are already using numerous resources for the management of disease symptoms and sequelae. An example is the long-term diabetic who requires costly revascularization procedures or experiences renal complications. With this group, episodic case management may have a small impact on cost and quality outcomes; even significant gains that can result from practice interventions may be of minimal impact on long-term outcomes.

The second subcategory includes those patients/members who have no active symptoms or complications that require immediate attention. The members of this group are typically active participants in their treatment regimens and have adequate self-management skills. Although this group would certainly be receptive to case management, education, or disease management strategies, case management may not yield the greatest return on investment, because these individuals are already actively engaged in preventive or effective health care behaviors.

Finally, a third subcategory of the chronic disease population includes those who are medically stable but have not adopted health care behaviors that limit disease progression and prevent serious complications. Such "passive participants," commonly referred to in the health care literature as being "noncompliant" or "nonadherent," may not engage in effective health care behaviors because of inability to access services, lack of education regarding the disease, or a clinician's failure to diagnose, prescribe, or coordinate. Additional reasons for "passive participation" may be related to depression, limited literacy skills, social isolation, economic constraints, cognitive disorders, lack of motivation, or conflicting health care beliefs. It is this population of "passive participants" who may yield the greatest return from appropriate case management intervention.

To achieve the greatest impact on costs in the most efficient manner, it is critical to target the high-utilization/expenditure groups within a larger population for early interventions to prevent complications or treat them promptly (Eichert, Wong, & Smith, 1997). A variety of methodologies may be used by the health care network or managed care organization to begin to sift through the larger population of enrollees in order to identify those individuals most amenable to case management. These include the use of the payer's claims data to identify those clients with various co-morbidities, diagnoses, or procedures.

Disease Management and the APN CM

Whether in a hospital or health plan environment, disease management strategies drive the care management team to control costs across the continuum and reduce long-term disease complications. Disease management has been described as a "proactive case management program" in which "the CM is accountable for cost-benefit and acuity management across the entire continuum" (Ward & Rieve, 1997, p. 256). However, an argument can be made that case management is a distinct strategy within the larger strategy of disease management. In this view, disease management may be seen as an organized process in which a community of health providers from many disciplines work together to ensure the appropriate management of a particular disease or population of patients. Although APN CMs may be instrumental in coordinating the efforts of a team developing such programs, they may simultaneously focus their case management practice within a specific point of care in the continuum. Thus, APN CMs collaborate with other providers to improve health care processes.

For example, one APN CM may work in the area of health promotion and disease prevention, assessing the population and developing longitudinal interventions to prevent costly debilitation associated with chronic disease in patients at risk. Another APN CM may practice in acute care and focus on complication management to achieve desired outcomes associated with hospital care. Finally, there are opportunities for the APN CM to practice within the community, following high-risk clients with pre-existing conditions, chronic disease, or terminal disease. At any point on the continuum, the APN CM may collaborate with physicians, NPs, and other providers to promote optimal treatment decisions and reduce costly variations among practitioners and health care delivery processes. The APN CM must have a working knowledge of all disease management system components including the people, the tools, and the evaluation methods.

Eichert and Patterson (1997) described the key elements of disease management as:

- Clinical management through the use of risk assessments and evidence-based guidelines
- Behavior modification through the application of theories and practices that apply to the particular population being managed for the specified disease
- Outcomes research for ongoing measurement that reflects behavior change, cost savings, and quality of clinical practice
- Financial management that can demonstrate cost of care across the continuum

In essence, the APN CM facilitates the development and implementation of a systematic approach to disease management that incorporates these elements for one or more points on the continuum of care.

Disease Management Interventions. Disease management interventions focus on behavior modification and outpatient activities. The APN CM addresses these components through staff education and team coordination. Whether the disease management program is for chronic low back pain, diabetes, multiple sclerosis, or congestive heart failure, the APN CM assumes a leadership role in establishing evidence-based practice guidelines and identifying appropriate patient interventions, such as telephone case management, selection of educational media for small group education/activities, or home visits. The intent of these interventions is to augment physician/NP visits and redirect care to an outpatient, less costly environment (Plocher, 1996).

Tools of Disease Management. It is essential to determine the appropriate vehicle to communicate the disease management strategy. APN CMs must be able to select the most effective tool to encourage an evidence-based approach to care. Is a critical pathway more practical than a care guideline? When is a protocol necessary? Would standardized medical orders guide the team to select recommended diagnostic and treatment practices? The APN CM needs to evaluate the process being altered and select the tool that will best guide decision making and influence clinical practice.

Disease Management Outcomes. The success of a disease management program is reflected in the following evaluation areas:

- Return on investment: How much did it cost to implement the program versus how much the organization saved during the period of time that the program was being evaluated?
- Changes in utilization patterns: Have admissions, readmission rates, or bed days/1,000 covered lives decreased significantly?
- Clinical outcomes: Is the diabetic patient staying within a desired range of glucose control as evidence by the hemoglobin A_1C blood test?
- Satisfaction of the patients, providers, and plans: Are patients more satisfied with their health, providers, and plans? Are the providers satisfied with their patients' health status and support services? Is the plan satisfied with the program? Did the disease management program demonstrate value for future marketing?

Looking Toward the Future of APN CM Practice

The future of APN CM practice will parallel the fluctuations in the health care arena. On the positive side, the APN CM may be the critical link in a continuum-based organization when it makes the transition from a predominantly fee-for-service model to a shared or global risk model. On the downside, many health care organizations are currently experiencing tremendous financial losses. As a result, many are returning to the "core business" of acute delivery and dramatically reducing resources once allotted to the continuum of care model.

Regulation and Credentialing

The health care provided by APNs has had far-reaching effects on members of society. However, with success come ever higher accountability and the need for more standardized ways to credential, certify, regulate, and sanction competent practice for a growing number of APNs. At both federal and state levels, this is a time of shifting priorities and changing models for nursing practice in all settings. It is an environment in which any discussion of regulatory issues is, by definition, fluid, dynamic, and subject to rapid change.

The challenge to provide standards of quality upon which advanced nursing practice can be framed, defended, and regulated is a serious one that requires constant attention. Issues involving education, scope of practice, specialty practice, reimbursement, and prescriptive authority are all embedded in regulatory language. To make the problem more difficult, regulatory issues are governed by multiple federal, state, educational, and professional entities whose work occurs in different venues, complicating efforts to collaborate (Hanson, 1998). It is important to understand that, for specific questions about up-to-the-minute, current APN rules and regulations, especially those that pertain to specific state statutes regarding ANP prescriptive authority and reimbursement, the reader is referred to individual local and state regulatory bodies for practice requirements.

The differences in education, certification, and individual scope of practice regulations from one advanced nursing specialty to another complicate issues for policy makers and regulators. Currently, the combined health care needs of an aging population, a period of economic retrenchment in health care, and the movement of both the public and private sectors of health care to a managed care environment have fostered a positive trend for advanced nursing practice. Health policy issues surrounding practice parameters, reimbursement, and choice of provider require careful consideration. All of these environmental phenomena have an impact, either directly, or indirectly, on the credentialing and regulatory policies that govern APN practice. Therefore, it is incumbent upon individual APNs to understand and practice within the parameters of these mechanisms.

When APNs seek to change statutes and regulations it is not because they see themselves as needing to practice in a vacuum of independence apart from the rest of the health care team. It is the challenge for APNs across the nation who are working to clarify statutory policies within state boards of nursing.

Scope of Practice for APNs

By definition, scope of practice describes practice limits and sets the parameters within which nurses in the various APN specialties may practice. Scope statements define what APNs can do for/with patients, what they can delegate, and when collaboration with others is required. Scope of practice statements tell APNs de facto what is beyond the limits of their nursing practice. Scope-of-practice statements are key to the debate about how the U.S. health care system uses APNs as health care providers; scope is inextricably linked with barriers to advanced nursing practice. The ability to diagnose and manage clients that is inherent to the role of the APN is fluid and evolving, and is in many instances tied to the collaborative relationships that APNs have with physician colleagues. It is important to understand that scope of practice differs from state to state and is based on state statutes promulgated by the various state nurse practice acts and the rules and regulations for APN practice.

Accountability becomes a crucial factor as APNs move toward authority over their own practices. Furthermore, it is crucial that scope-of-practice statements that are presented by national certifying entities are carried through in scope-of-practice language in state statutes.

The American Nurses Association's (ANA's) definition of an APN requires that the role be clinically focused and that the APN give direct clinical care to patients. This designation of what constitutes an APN is primarily driven by two factors: the ability for APNs to be directly reimbursed and the degree to which nurses desire prescriptive and admitting privileges. The reason for this clear definition is that there must be an efficacious way for state boards, insurers, prescribing entities, and the like to monitor the scope of practice, prescribing, and reimbursement patterns of APNs. There is an ongoing dialogue between national certifying bodies and state regulators, as well as among bodies who accredit educational programs, to bring standardization to the multiple APN specialties.

Implications of Standards of Practice and Standard of Care for APNs

Standards of practice for nursing are defined by the profession nationally and help to further explicate and delineate scope of practice. Standards are overarching, authoritative statements that the nursing profession uses to describe the responsibilities for which its members are accountable (ANA, 1996). APNs are held to both the standards of practice promulgated by the nursing profession and to standards of the various APN specialties. At both levels, standards of practice describe the basic competency levels for safe and competent practice. Professional standards of practice match closely with the core competencies for APNs that undergird advanced nursing practice.

Standards of care differ from the standards of practice set forth by the nursing profession. These standards are often termed "practice guidelines." Practice guidelines provide a foundation by which health care providers administer care to patients. These guidelines crosscut the health professions' disciplines and are the frameworks/standards by which basic safety and competent care are measured. Standards of care are derived from evidence-based practice and are evolving over time. It is very important that APNs are part of interdisciplinary teams that develop and test practice guidelines for care.

Legal Concerns Surrounding Advanced Nursing Practice

There are several reasons why the multiplicity of titles and roles for APNs is a problem from a policy viewpoint. The first and foremost reason is that it is confusing to policy makers and regulators. It is especially a problem at agencies such as the Health Care Financing Agency, where major designations for Medicare and Medicaid reimbursement set the standard for all reimbursement across the country. In addition, discrepancies among states make mobility difficult for APNs in terms of prescriptive authority and reimbursement.

APNs are primarily responsible to and are disciplined by individual state boards of nursing. One of the licensing and credentialing difficulties faced by APNs is the variance in board regulations from state to state. In some states APN practice is governed solely by the board of nursing; in others it is jointly administered by the boards of nursing and medicine; and in still others it is governed by the boards of nursing and pharmacy. As APNs move in and out of what is considered the domain of medicine, serious thought must be given to the standard by which APNs will be judged if they are deemed to have made an error. It is incumbent upon APNs to set clear standards for practice that are based on clinical competency.

APN Credentialing and Regulation

"Credentialing" is an umbrella term that refers to the regulatory mechanisms that can be applied to individuals, programs, or organizations (Styles, 1998). APN program accreditation and approval, scope of practice, standards of practice, practice guidelines, and collaborative practice agreements all have important implications for APNs in terms of proper credentialing and interactions with the court system. These documents create the standard by which APN practice is monitored and regulated, deemed safe or unsafe, and by which APNs are disciplined from state to state.

State Licensure/Recognition as a Component of APN Credentialing

State law that provides oversight to APN practice is divided into two forms: statutes as defined by the nurse practice act enacted by the state legislature, and rules and regulations explicated by state agencies under the jurisdiction of the executive branch of state government (Buppert, 1999). Licensure is the authority delegated to the individual states by the federal Constitution, which provides standards to assure basic levels of public safety. In most states, the board of nursing has sole authority over APN practice; however, in 11 states there is joint authority with the board of medicine (Buppert, 1999). The states require that all APNs carry current licensure as an RN. Advanced nursing practice status is achieved through rules and regulations that are part of the individual state nurse practice act. Authority to practice is tied to scope of practice and varies from state to state depending on the degree of practice autonomy the APN is granted. Most states require national certification and proof of completion of an approved APN program. Pharmacology requirements vary from state to state, although currently most states require a graduate core pharmacotherapeutics course during the APN educational program and yearly continuing education (CE) credits thereafter to maintain prescriptive privileges.

Credentialing/licensure for prescriptive authority occurs at the state level. The process varies from state to state depending on how the statute is written. Prescribing authority may be regulated solely by the board of nursing, as it is in several states; jointly by the board of nursing and the board of pharmacy, as it is in several others; or by a triad of boards of nursing, medicine, and pharmacy. It is incumbent upon the APN to clearly understand the mechanisms whereby prescriptive authority is regulated in a given state.

As prescriptive authority has evolved over the past several years, certain basic requirements have become fairly (although not entirely) standard for APN prescribers. They are as follows:

1. Graduation from an approved master's level APN program
2. Licensure/recognition in good standing as an APN
3. National certification in an APN specialty
4. A recent pharmacotherapeutics course of at least 3 credit hours (45 contact hours)
5. Evidence of a collaborative practice arrangement (in some states)
6. Ongoing CE hours in pharmacotherapeutics to maintain prescribing status
7. State prescribing and national Drug Enforcement Administration numbers in some instances
8. A pharmacy formulary (in some states)

These requirements vary from state to state but provide a core regulatory process for prescriptive authority (Buppert, 1999; Hanson, 1996).

National Certification as a Component of APN Credentialing

National Certification.   National certification for APNs, over time, has served several purposes, including regulation and licensure, entry into practice, validation of competence, and a way to recognize expert practice (Lewis, Camp, & Rothrock, 1996). Multiple bodies for certification have surfaced to fill the need for APN certification, which has resulted in varying certification requirements (Hodnicki, 1998). APN certification is national in scope and is a mandatory requirement for APNs to obtain and maintain credentialing in most but not all states (Pearson, 2000). More and more state regulatory bodies are currently using national certification examinations as a component of the credentialing mechanism.

Recertification. Overall, APNs must fulfill CE and practice requirements to successfully maintain their national certification, although differences in requirements exist from specialty to specialty. Each APN certification entity clearly lays out the requirements and time frame for recertification. Generally, national certification for most specialties lasts from 5 to 8 years and requires that the candidate retest unless the established parameters are met.

Mandatory Practice Requirements. Most, but not all, APN specialties have built in specific requirements for an adequate number of clinical practice hours between the years of recertification to assure that APNs are maintaining currency and competence through regular practice as an APN. APNs who do not meet stipulated CE and practice requirements must retake the national certifying board exam to continue to practice. National certification assures national consistency of professional standards and helps the public to understand the APN scope of practice (AACN, 1995). It is one way to assure that competent APNs provide needed health care to patients and families. Therefore, standardization of APN certification and recertification processes is critical in order to assure the credibility of APN specialties (Hodnicki, 1998).

Collaborative Practice Arrangements

The general term "practice guidelines" can be confusing to the APN in that it is used in several different contexts. First, it is an evidence-based standard of care. However, it is also used to refer to a collegial agreement between the APN and the physician to define parameters of practice for the APN. Collegial practice agreements take many forms, from a one-page written agreement defining consultation and referral patterns to a more specific prescribed "protocol" for specific functions. The term "protocol" in relation to advanced nursing practice was common several years ago as a directed, specified guideline for practice that defined each patient problem and the care directive.

The norm today in APN regulation is shifting towards loosely configured collaborative relationships that offer support to all parties and protect the safety of patients. Collaborative relationships vary widely from APN specialty to specialty.

Institutional Credentialing

The need for hospital privileges for APNs varies according to the nurse's practice. For example, CNMs and many rural NPs cannot properly care for patients without the ability to admit to the hospital should the need arise. The rules for practice as part of the hospital staff are even more specific and variable than those for prescriptive authority and are bound to the local hospital or medical facility and the medical staff of the granting institution.

Future Regulatory Challenges Facing APNs

"Certification is a form of credentialing and credentialing is a form of regulation" (Styles, 1998). At no time has it been more important that APNs understand and value the important relationships that underpin the complex processes and systems that regulate practice. New models of health care and varying configurations of how APNs practice in interdisciplinary teams escalates the importance of regulatory considerations to new levels.

References

Ad Hoc Committee on Health Literacy for the Council on Scientific Affairs, American Medical Association. (1999). Health literacy: Report of the Council on Scientific Affairs. *JAMA, 281,* 552-557.

Ahronheim, J.C., Moreno, J., & Zuckerman, C. (1994). *Ethics in clinical practice.* Boston: Little, Brown.

Alpert, H., Goldman, L., Kilroy, C., & Pike, A. (1992). 7 Gryzmish: Toward an understanding of collaboration. *Nursing Clinics of North America, 27,* 47-59.

American Association of Colleges of Nursing. (1995). *The essentials of master's education for advanced practice nursing.* Washington, DC: Author.

American Nurses Association. (1980). *Nursing: A social policy statement.* Kansas City, MO: Author.

American Nurses Association. (1995). *Nursing's social policy statement.* Washington, DC: Author.

American Nurses Association. (1996). *Scope and standards of advanced practice registered nursing.* Washington, DC: Author.

Arena, D.M., & Page, N.E. (1992). The imposter phenomenon in the clinical nurse specialist role. *Image: The Journal of Nursing Scholarship, 24*(2), 121-125.

Aroskar, M. (1998). Ethical working relationships in patient care. *Nursing Clinics in North America, 33*(2), 313-324.

Arslanian-Engoren, C.M. (1995). Lived experiences of CNSs who collaborate with physicians: A phenomenological study. *Clinical Nurse Specialist, 9*(2), 68-73.

Baggs, J.G., & Schmitt. M.C. (1988). Collaboration between nurses and physicians. *Image: The Journal of Nursing Scholarship, 20,* 145-149.

Baird, S.B., & Prouty, M.P. (1989). In A.B. Hamric & J.A. Spross (Eds.), *The clinical nurse specialist in theory and practice* (2nd ed., pp. 261-284). Philadelphia: W.B. Saunders.

Ballein, K.M. (1998). Entrepreneurial leadership characteristics of SNEs emerge as their role develops. *Nursing Administration Quarterly, 22*(2), 60-69.

Barnason, S., Merboth, M., Pozehl, B., & Tietjen, M.J. (1998). Utilizing an outcome approach to improve pain management by nurses: A pilot study. *Clinical Nurse Specialist, 12*(1), 28-36.

Barron, A.-M. (1989). The clinical nurse specialist as consultant. In A.B. Hamric & J.A. Spross (Eds.), *The clinical nurse specialist in theory and practice* (2nd ed., pp. 125-146). Philadelphia: W.B. Saunders.

Barron, A.-M., & White, P. (1996). Consultation. In A.B. Hamric, J.A. Spross, & C.M. Hanson (Eds.), *Advanced nursing practice: An integrative approach* (pp. 165-183). Philadelphia: W.B. Saunders.

Beare, P.G. (1989). The essentials of win-win negotiation for the clinical nurse specialist. *Clinical Nurse Specialist, 13*(3), 138.

Beauchamp, T.L., & Childress, J.F. (1994). *Principles of biomedical ethics* (4th ed.). New York: Oxford University Press.

Benner, P. (1985). The oncology clinical nurse specialist as expert coach. *Oncology Nursing Forum, 12*(2), 40-44.

Benner, P. (1991). The role of experience, narrative and community in skilled ethical comportment. *Advances in Nursing Science, 14*(2), 1.

Benner, P., Hooper-Kyriakidis, P., & Stannard, D. (1999). *Clinical wisdom and interventions in critical care: A thinking-in-action approach.* Philadelphia: W.B. Saunders.

Benner, P., Tanner, C.A. & Chesla, C.A. (1996). *Expertise in Nursing Practice: Caring, clinical judgment and ethics.* New York: Springer-Verlag.

Boyle, D. McC. (1996). The clinical nurse specialist. In A.B. Hamric, J.A. Spross, & C.M. Hanson (Eds.), *Advanced nursing practice: An integrative approach* (pp. 299-336). Philadelphia: W.B. Saunders.

Bridges, W. (1991). Managing transitions: Making the most of change. Reading, MA: Addison-Wesley.

Brooten, D., Gennaro, S., Knapp, H., Jovene, N., Brown, L., & York, R. (1991). Functions of the CNS in early discharge and home follow-up of very low birthweight infants. *Clinical Nurse Specialist, 5*(4), 196-201.

Brooten, D., Kumer, S., Brown, L.P., Butts, P., Finkler, S.A., Bakewell-Sachs, S., Gibbons, A., & Delivoria-Papadopoulos, M. (1986). A randomized clinical trial of early hospital discharge and home follow-up of very-low-birth-weight infants. *New England Journal of Medicine, 315*(15), 934-939.

Brooten, D., & Naylor, M.D. (1995). Nurses' effect on changing patient outcomes. *Image: The Journal of Nursing Scholarship, 27*(2), 95-99.

Brooten, D., Roncoli, M., Finkler, S., Arnold, L., Cohen, A., & Menuti, M. (1994). A randomized trial of early hospital discharge and home follow-up of women having cesarean birth. *Obstetrics and Gynecology, 84*(5), 832-838.

Broussard, B.S. (1996). The role of the perinatal home care clinical nurse specialist. *Home Healthcare Nurse, 14*(11), 855-860.

Brown, M.A., & Olshansky, E. (1998). Becoming a primary care nurse practitioner: Challenges of the initial year of practice. *Nurse Practitioner, 23*(7), 46, 52-58, 61-66.

Brown, M.A., & Olshansky, E.F. (1997). From limbo to legitimacy: A theoretical model of the transition to the primary care nurse practitioner role. *Nursing Research, 46*(1), 46-51.

Brown, S.J. (1998). A framework for advanced practice nursing. *Journal of Professional Nursing, 14*(3), 157-164.

Brown, S.J. (1999). Knowledge for health care practice: A guide to using research evidence. Philadelphia: W.B. Saunders.

Brown, S.J. (1989). Supportive supervision of the CNS. In A.B. Hamric & J.A. Spross (Eds.), *The clinical nurse specialist in theory and practice* (2nd ed., pp. 285-298). Philadelphia: W.B. Saunders.

Brykczynski, K.A. (1989). An interpretive study describing the clinical judgement of nurse practitioners. *Scholarly Inquiry for Nursing Practice, 3,* 75-104.

Brykczynski, K.A. (1996). Role development of the advanced practice nurse. In A.B. Hamric, J.A. Spross, & C.M. Hanson (Eds.), *Advanced nursing practice: An integrative approach* (pp. 89-95). Philadelphia: W.B. Saunders.

Brykczynski, K.A. (1991). Judgement strategies for coping with ambiguous clinical situations encountered in primary family care. *Journal of the American Academy of Nurse Practitioners, 3*(2), 79-84.

Bulechek, G.M., & McCloskey, J.C. (1999a). Nursing diagnoses, interventions, and outcomes in effectiveness research. In G.M. Bulechek & J.C. McCloskey (Eds.), *Nursing interventions classification: Effective nursing treatments* (3rd ed., pp. 1-26). Philadelphia: W.B. Saunders.

Buppert, C. (1999). Nurse practitioner's business practice and legal guide. Gaithersburg, MD: Aspen Publishers.

Burns, J.M. (1978). *Leadership.* New York: Harper & Row.

Calkin, J.D. (1984). A model for advanced nursing practice. *Journal of Nursing Administration, 14*(1), 24-30.

Calkins, M.E. (1993). Ethical issues in the elderly ESRD patient. *ANNA Journal, 20*(5), 569.

Caplan, G. (1970). The theory and practice of mental health consultation. New York: Basic Books.

Caplan, G., & Caplan, R. (1993). *Mental health consultation and collaboration.* San Francisco: Jossey-Bass.

Case Management Society of America. (1994). CMSA proposes standards of practice. *The Case Manager, 5*(1), 59-70.

Chase, L.K., Johnson, S.K., Laffoon, T.A., Jacobs, R.S., & Johnson, M.E. (1996). CNS role: An experience in retitling and role clarification. *Clinical Nurse Specialist, 10*(1), 41-45.

Chick, N., & Meleis, A. (1986). Transitions: A nursing concern. In P. Chinn (Ed.), *Nursing research methodology: Issues and implementation* (pp. 237-258). Rockville, MD: Aspen Publishers.

Childress, J.F. (1994). Principles-oriented bioethics: An analysis and assessment from within. In E.R. DuBose, R. Hamel, & L.J. O'Connell (Eds.), *A matter of principles?* (pp. 72-98). Valley Forge, PA: Trinity Press International.

Clarke, E.B. & Spross, J.A. (1996). Expert coaching and guidance. In A.B. Hamric, J.A. Spross, & C.M. Hanson (Eds.), *Advanced nursing practice: An integrative approach* (pp. 139-164). Philadelphia: W.B. Saunders.

Colman, N.S. (1992). Variability in consultation rates and practitioner level of diagnostic certainty. *Journal of Family Practice, 35*(1), 31-38.

Connelly, C. (1993). An empirical model of self-care in chronic illness. *Clinical Nurse Specialist, 7,* 247-253.

Connors, H. (1993). Impact of care management modalities on curricula. In K. Kelly & M. Maas (Eds.), *Managing nursing care: Promise and pitfalls* (pp. 190-207). St. Louis: Mosby.

Cooper, D.M. (1990). Today - assessment and intuition: Tomorrow - projections. In D.M. Cooper, P.A. Minarik, & P.S.A. Sparacino (Eds.), *The clinical nurse specialist: Implementation and impact* (pp. 285-298). Norwalk, CT: Appleton & Lange.

Cooper, D.M., & Sparacino, P.S.A. (1990). Acquiring, implementing, and evaluating the clinical nurse specialist role. In P.S.A. Sparacino, D.M. Copper, & P.A. Minarik (Eds.), *The clinical nurse specialist: Implementation and impact* (pp. 41-75). Norwalk, CT: Appleton & Lange.

Cooper, M.C. (1989). Gilligan's different voice: A perspective for nursing. *Journal of Professional Nursing, 5*(1), 10-16.

Cooper, R.A., Henderson, T., & Dietrich, C.L. (1998). Roles of nonphysician clinicians as autonomous providers in patient care. *JAMA, 280,* 795-800.

Cooper-Patrick, L., Gallo, J.J., Gonzales, J.J., Vu, H.T., Powe, N.R., & Ford, D.E. (1999). Race, gender, and partnership in the patient-physician relationship. *JAMA, 282,* 583-589.

Copp, L.A. (1986). The nurse as an advocate for vulnerable persons. *Journal of Advanced Nursing, 11*(3), 255-263.

Corbin, J., & Strauss, A. (1992). A nursing model for chronic illness management based upon the trajectory framework. In P. Woog (Ed.), *The chronic illness trajectory framework: The Corbin and Strauss model* (pp. 9-28). New York: Springer-Verlag.

Covey, S. (1989). The seven habits of highly effective people: Powerful lessons in personal change. New York: Simon & Schuster.

Cronenwett, L.R. (1995). Modeling the future of advanced practice nursing. *Nursing Outlook, 43,* 112-118.

Damato, E.G., Dill, P.Z., Gennaro, S., Brown, L.P., York, R., & Brooten, D. (1993). The association between CNS direct care time and total time and very low birth weight infant outcomes. *Clinical Nurse Specialist, 7,* 75-79.

Davies, B., & Hughes, A.M. (1995). Clarification of advanced nursing practice: Characteristics and competencies. *Clinical Nurse Specialist, 9,* 156-160.

Deaton, C. (1998a). Outcomes measurement. *Journal of Cardiovascular Nursing, 12*(4), 49-51.

Deaton, C. (1998b). Outcomes measurement: Multidisciplinary approaches and patient outcomes after stroke. *Journal of Cardiovascular Nursing, 13*(1), 93-96.

Dreyfus, H.L., & Dreyfus, S.E. (1977). *Uses and abuses of multi-attribute and multi-aspect model of decision making.* Unpublished manuscript, Department of Industrial Engineering and Operations Research, University of California at Berkeley.

Dreyfus, H.L., & Dreyfus, S.E. (1986). Mind over machine: The power of human intuition and expertise in the era of the computer. New York: Free Press.

Eichert, J.H., & Patterson, R.B. (1997). Factors affecting the success of disease management. *Infusion, 3*(12), 31-38.

Eichert, J.H., Wong, H., & Smith, D.R. (1997). The disease management development process. In W.E. Todd & D. Nash (Eds.), *Disease management: A system approach to improving patient outcomes* (pp. 27-60). Chicago: American Hospital Publishing.

Erickson, H.C., Tomlin, E.M., & Swain, M.P. (1983). *Modeling and role-modeling: A theory and paradigm for nursing.* Englewood Cliffs, NJ: Prentice Hall.

Evans, J.A. (1994). The role of the nurse manager in creating an environment for collaborative practice. *Holistic Nursing Practice, 8*(3), 23-31.

Evidence-Based Working Group. (1992). Evidence based medicine: A new approach to teaching the practice of medicine. *JAMA, 268,* 2420-2425.

Fagin, C. (1992). Collaboration between nurses and physicians: No longer a choice. *Nursing and Health Care, 13,* 354-363.

Fagin, C.M. (1998). Nursing research and the erosion of care. *Nursing Outlook, 46*(6), 259-260.

Fenton, M.V. (1985). Identifying competencies of clinical nurse specialists. *Journal of Nursing Administration, 15*(12), 31-37.

Fenton, M.V, & Brykczynski, K.A. (1993). Qualitative distinctions and similarities in the practice of clinical nurse specialists and nurse practitioners. *Journal of Professional Nursing, 9,* 313-326.

Fisher, R., & Ury, W. (1981). *Getting to yes.* New York: Viking Penguin.

Forbes, E., & Fitzsimmons, V. (1993). Education: The key for holistic interdisciplinary collaboration. *Holistic Nursing Practice, 7*(4), 1-10.

Forrow, L., Arnold, R.M., & Parker, L.S. (1993). Preventive ethics: Expanding the horizons of clinical ethics. *Journal of Clinical Ethics 4*(4), 287-294.

Fralic, M. (1992). The nurse case manager: Focus, selection, preparation, and measurement. *Journal of Nursing Administration, 22*(11), 13-14, 46.

Frisch, M., Elliott, C., Atsaides, J., Salva, D., & Denney, D. (1982). Social skills and stress management training to enhance patients' interpersonal competencies. *Psychotherapy Theory, Research and Practice, 19,* 349-358.

Gaul, A.L. (1995). Casuistry, care, compassion and ethics data analysis. *Advances in Nursing Science, 17*(3), 47.

Gianakos, D. (1997). Physicians, nurses and collegiality. *Nursing Outlook, 45*(2), 57-58.

Gilligan, C. (1982). *In a different voice.* Cambridge, MA: Harvard University Press.

Girouard, S. (1983). Theory-based practice: Functions, obstacles, and solutions. In A.B. Hamric & J.A. Spross (Eds.), *The clinical nurse specialist in theory and practice* (pp. 21-37). New York: Grune & Stratton.

Girouad, S.A. (1996). Evaluating advanced nursing practice. In A.B. Hamric, J.A. Spross, & C.M. Hanson (Eds.), *Advanced nursing practice: An integrative approach* (pp. 569-600). Philadelphia: W.B. Saunders.

Gordon, M., Murphy, C.P., Candee, D., & Hiltunen, E. (1994). Clinical judgement: An integrated model. *Advances in Nursing Science, 16,* 55-70.

Grumbach, K., & Coffman, J. (1998). Physicians and nonphysician clinicians. *JAMA, 280,* 825-826.

Gudorf, C.E. (1994). A feminist critique of biomedical principlism. In E.R. DuBose, R. Hamel, & L.J. O'Connell (Eds.), *A matter of principles?* (pp. 164-181). Valley Forge, PA: Trinity Press International.

Hamric, A.B. (1983). Role development and functions. In A.B. Hamric & J. Spross (Eds.), *The clinical nurse specialist in theory and practice* (pp. 39-56). New York: Grune & Stratton.

Hamric, A.B. (1989a). History and overview of the CNS role. In A.B. Hamric & J.A. Spross (Eds.), *The clinical nurse specialist in theory and practice* (2nd ed., pp. 3-18). Philadelphia: W.B. Saunders.

Hamric, A.B. (1989b). A model for CNS evaluation. In A.B. Hamric & J.A. Spross (Eds.), *The clinical nurse specialist in theory and practice* (2nd ed., pp. 83-104). Philadelphia: W.B. Saunders.

Hamric, A.B. (1992). Creating our future: Challenges and opportunities for the clinical nurse specialist. *Oncology Nursing Forum, 19*(1, Suppl), 11-15.

Hamric, A.B., & Spross, J.A. (Eds.). (1989). *The clinical nurse specialist in theory and practice* (2nd ed.). Philadelphia: W.B. Saunders.

Hamric, A.B., Spross, J.A., & Hanson, C.M. (1996). *Advanced nursing practice: An integrative approach.* Philadelphia: W.B. Saunders.

Hamric, A.B., & Taylor, J.W. (1989). Role development of the CNS. In A.B. Hamric & J. Spross (Eds.), *The clinical nurse specialist in theory and practice* (2nd ed., pp. 41-82). Philadelphia: W.B. Saunders.

Hanson, C.M. (1996). Health policy issues: Dealing with the realities and constraints of advanced practice nursing. In A.B. Hamric, J.A. Spross, & C.M. Hanson (Eds.), *Advanced nursing practice: An integrative approach* (pp. 496-515). Philadelphia: W.B. Saunders.

Hanson, C.M. (1998). Regulatory issues will lead advanced practice nursing challenges into the new millennium. *Advanced Practice Nursing Quarterly, 4*(3), v-vi.

Hanson, J.L., & Ashley, B. (1994). Advanced practice nurses' application of the Stetler Model for Research Utilization: Improving bereavement care. *Oncology Nursing Forum, 21,* 720-724.

Hardy, M.E., & Hardy, W.L. (1988). Role stress and role strain. In M.E. Hardy & M.E. Conway (Eds.), *Role theory: Perspectives for health professionals* (2nd ed., pp. 159-239). Norwalk, CT: Appleton & Lange.

Harris, M. (1997). Reduced risk of complex response: An invisible outcome. *Nursing Administration Quarterly, 21*(4), 25-31.

Hickey, M. (1990). The role of the clinical nurse specialist in the research utilization process. *Clinical Nurse Specialist, 4,* 93-96.

Hodgman, E.C. (1983). The CNS as researcher. In A.B. Hamric & J.A. Spross (Eds.), *The clinical nurse specialist in theory and practice* (pp. 73-82). New York: Grune & Stratton.

Hodnicki, D.R. (1998). Advanced practice nursing certification: Where do we go from here? *Advanced Practice Nursing Quarterly, 4*(3), 34-43.

Hops, H. (1983). Children's social competence and skill: Current research, practices, and future directions. *Behavioral Therapy, 14,* 3-18.

Houston, S., & Luquire, R. (1997). Advanced practice nurse as outcomes manager. *Advanced Practice Nursing Quarterly, 3*(2), 1-9.

Hughes, A., & Mackenzie, C. (1990). Components necessary in a successful nurse practitioner-physician collaborative practice. *Journal of the American Academy of Nurse Practitioners, 2*(2), 54-57.

Inglis, A., & Kjervik, D. (1993). Empowerment of advanced practice nurses: Regulation reform needed to increase access to care. *Journal of Law, Medicine & Ethics, 21*(2), 193-205.

Jenny, J., & Logan, J. (1992). Knowing the patient: One aspect of clinical knowledge. *Image: The Journal of Nursing Scholarship, 24,* 254-258.

Jonsen, A.R., & Toulmin, S. (1988). *The abuse of casuistry: A history of moral reasoning.* Berkeley: University of California Press.

Kantor, R.M., Stein, B.A., & Jick, T.D. (1992). The challenge of organizational change: How companies experience it and leaders guide it. New York: The Free Press.

Kasch, C., & Dine, J. (1988). Person-centered communication and social perspective taking. *Western Journal of Nursing Research, 10,* 317-326.

Kibbe, D.C. (1999, March). Best practice interview: David C. Kibbe. http://ww1.best4health.org/resources/interviews/interview-kibbe.cfm

Kirsch, I., Jungeblut, A., Jenkins, L., & Kolstad, A. (1993). *Adult literacy in America: A first look at the findings of the National Adult Literacy Survey.* Washington, DC: U.S. Department of Education, National Center for Education Statistics.

Klein, E., Gabelnick, F., & Herr, P. (1998). *The psychodynamics of leadership.* Madison, CT: Psychosocial Press.

Koetters, T.L. (1989). Clinical practice and direct patient care. In A.B. Hamric & J.A. Spross (Eds.), *The clinical nurse specialist in theory and practice* (2nd ed., pp. 107-124). Philadelphia: W.B. Saunders.

Koetters, T.L. (1989). Clinical practice and direct patient care. In A.B. Hamric & J.A. Spross (Eds.), *The clinical nurse specialist in theory and practice* (2nd ed., pp. 107-124). Philadelphia: W.B. Saunders.

Kolcaba, K. (1992). Holistic comfort: Operationalizing the construct as a nurse-sensitive outcome. *Advances in Nursing Science, 15*(1), 1-10.

Krouse, H.J., & Roberts, S.J. (1989). Nurse-patient interactive styles: Power, control, and satisfaction. *Western Journal of Nursing Research, 11*(6) 717-725.

Krumm, S. (1992). Collaboration between oncology clinical nurse specialists and nursing administrators. *Oncology Nursing Forum, 19*(1, Suppl.), 21-24.

LaMear-Tucker, D., & Friedson, J. (1997). Resolving moral conflict: The critical care nurses' role. *Critical Care Nurse, 17*(2), 55.

Lang, N., & Marek, K. (1992). Outcomes that reflect clinical practice. In *Patient outcomes research: Examining the effectiveness of nursing practice* (NIH Publication No. 93-3411) (pp. 27-38). Rockville, MD: National Institutes of Health.

Larson, E. (1999). The impact of physician-nurse interaction on patient care. *Holistic Nursing Practice, 13*(2), 38-46.

Lewin, K. (1951). *Field theory in social science.* New York: Harper & Row.

Lewis, C.K., Camp, J., & Rothrock, J. (1996). The Trilateral Initiative for North American Nursing: Nursing specialty certification in the United States. An assessment of North American nursing. Philadelphia: Commission on Graduates of Foreign Nursing Schools.

Lindeke, L.L., & Block, D.E. (1998). Maintaining professional integrity in the midst of interdisciplinary collaboration. *Nursing Outlook, 46,* 213-218.

Lipowski, Z.J. (1981). Liaison psychiatry, liaison nursing and behavioral medicine. *Comprehensive Psychiatry, 22,* 554-561.

Lynch, V.A. (1991). Forensic nursing in the emergency department: A new role for the 1990's. *Critical Care Nursing Quarterly, 14*(3), 69-86.

Mackay, M.H. (1998). Research utilization and the CNS: Confronting the issues. *Clinical Nurse Specialist, 12,* 232-237.

Mahn, V.A., & Spross, J.A. (1996). Nurse case management as an advanced practice role. In A.B. Hamric, J.A. Spross, & C.M. Hanson (Eds.), *Advanced nursing practice: An integrative approach* (pp. 445-465). Philadelphia: W.B. Saunders.

Martocchio, B. (1987). Authenticity, belonging, emotional closeness, and self representation. *Oncology Nursing Forum, 14*(4), 23-27.

Mathew, L.J., Gutsch, H.M., Hackney, N.W. & Munsat, E.M. (1994). Promoting quality and cost-effective care to geropsychiatric patients. *Issues in Mental Health Nursing, 15*(2), 169-185.

McAlpine, L.A. (1997). Process and outcome measures for the multidisciplinary collaborative projects of a critical care CNS. *Clinical Nurse Specialist, 11*(3), 134-138.

McGuire, D.B. (1992, January). *The process of implementing research into clinical practice.* (Publication No. 92-50M-No. 3350.00-PE. Proceedings of the American Cancer Society Second National Conference on Cancer Nursing Research). Atlanta: American Cancer Society.

McGuire, D.B., & Harwood, K.V. (1989). The CNS as researcher. In A.B. Hamric & J.A. Spross (Eds.), *The clinical nurse specialist in theory and practice* (2nd ed., pp. 169-204). Philadelphia: W.B. Saunders.

McGuire, D.B., & Harwood, K.V. (1996). Research implementation, utilization, and conduct. In A.B. Hamric, J.A. Spross, & C.M. Hanson (Eds.), *Advanced nursing practice: An integrative approach* (pp. 184-212). Philadelphia: W.B. Saunders.

McGuire, D.B., DeLoney, V.G., Yeager, K.A., Owen, D.C., Peterson, D.E., Lin, L.S., & Webster, J. (2000). Maintaining study validity in a changing clinical environment. *Nursing Research.*

McPheeters, M., & Lohr, K.N. (1999). Evidence-based practice and nursing: Commentary. *Outcomes Management for Nursing Practice, 3*(3), 99-101.

Minarik, P.A., & Sparacino, P.S.A. (1990). Clinical nurse specialist collaboration in a university medical center. In P.S.A. Sparacino, D.M. Cooper, & P.A. Minarik (Eds.), *The clinical nurse specialist: Implementation and impact* (pp. 231-260). East Norwalk, CT: Appleton & Lange.

Mitchell, P.H., & Shortell, S.M. (1997). Adverse outcomes and variation in organization of care delivery. *Medical Care, 35,* 19-32.

Mitchell, P.H., Ferketich, S., & Jennings, B.M. (1998). Quality health outcomes model. *Image: The Journal of Nursing Scholarship, 30*(1), 43-46.

Montgomery, C.L. (1993). *Healing through communication.* Newbury Park, CA: Sage Publications.

Mundinger, M.O., Kane, R.L., Lenz, E.R., Totten, A.M., Tsai, W.-Y., Cleary, P.D., Friedewald, W.T., Siu, A.L., & Shelanski, M.L. (2000). Primary care outcomes in patients treated by nurse practitioners or physicians: A randomized trial. *Jama, 283,* 59-68.

Narayan, S.M., & Corcoran-Perry, S. (1997). Line of reasoning as a representation of nurses' clinical decision making. *Research in Nursing and Health, 20,* 353-364.

National Association of Clinical Nurse Specialists. (1998). *Statement on clinical nurse specialist practice and education.* Glenview, IL: Author.

National Council of State Boards of Nursing. (1998). *Interstate compact for a mutual recognition model of nursing.* Chicago: Author.

National Organization of Nurse Practitioner Faculties. (1995). Advanced nursing practice: Curriculum guidelines and program standards for nurse practitioner education. Washington, DC: Author.

Naylor, M., Brooten, D., Campbell, R., Jacobsen, B.S., Mezey, M.D., Pauly, M.V., & Schwartz, J.S. (1999). Comprehensive discharge planning and home follow-up of hospitalized elders. *JAMA, 281,* 613-657.

Naylor, M., Brooten, D., Jones, R., Lavizzo-Mourey, R., Mezey, M., & Pauly, M. (1994). Comprehensive discharge planning for the hospitalized elderly. A randomized trial. *Annals of Internal Medicine, 120,* 999-1006.

Naylor, M., Munro, B., & Brooten, D. (1991). Measuring the effectiveness of nursing practice. *Clinical Nurse Specialist, 5,* 210-215.

Neidinger, S., Kennedy, L., & Scroggins, K. (1987). Effective and cost efficient discharge planning for hospitalized elders. *Nursing economics, 5*(5), 225-230.

Nelson, E.C., Splaine, M.E., Batalden, P.B., & Plume, S.K. (1998). Building measurement and data collection into medical practice. *Annals of Internal Medicine, 128,* 460-466.

Newman, M. (1990). Toward an integrative model of professional practice. *Journal of Professional Nursing, 6,* 167-173.

Norwood, S.L. (1998). When the CNS needs a consultant. *Clinical Nurse Specialist, 12,* 53-58.

Nugent, K.E., & Lambert, V.A. (1996). The advanced practice nurse in collaborative practice. *Nursing Connections, 9*(1), 5-14.

Oddi, L.F. & Cassidy, V.R. (1998). The message of SUPPORT: Change is long overdue. *Journal of Professional Nursing, 14*(3), 165-174.

Office of Technology Assessment. (1986). *Nurse practitioners, physician assistants, and certified nurse midwives: A policy analysis* (Health Care Technology Study No. OTA-HCS-37). Washington, DC: Author.

Olczak, P.V., Grosch, J.W., & Duffy, K.G. (1991). Toward a synthesis: The art with the science of community mediation. In K.G. Duffy, J.W. Grosch, & P.V. Olczak (Eds.), *Community mediation* (pp. 329-343). New York: The Guilford Press.

Olesen, V., Schatzman, L., Droes, N., Hatton, D., & Chico, N. (1990). The mundane ailment and the physical self: Analysis of the social psychology of health and illness. *Social Science and Medicine, 30,* 449-455.

Omery, A., Henneman, E., Billet, B., Luna-Raines, M., & Brown-Saltzman, K. (1995). Ethical issues in hospital-based nursing practice. *Journal of Cardiovascular Nursing, 9*(3), 43-53.

O'Neill, E.S. (1995). Heuristics reasoning in diagnostic judgement. *Journal of Professional Nursing, 11,* 239-245.

Ostermeyer, M. (1991). Conducting the mediation. In K.G. Duffy, J.W. Grosch, & P.V. Olczak (Eds.), *Community mediation* (pp. 91-104). New York: The Guilford Press.

Payne, J.L., & Baumgartner, R.G. (1996). CNS role evolution. *Clinical Nurse Specialist, 10*(1), 46-48.

Pearson, L. (2000). Annual update of how each state stands on legislative issues affecting advanced nursing practice. *The Nurse Practitioner: The American Journal of Primary Health Care, 25*(1), 16-68.

Pellegrino, E.D. (1996). What's wrong with the nurse-physician relationship in today's hospitals? A physician's view. *Hospitals, 40,* 70-80.

Pelligrini, D., & Urbain, E. (1985). An evaluation of interpersonal cognitive problem solving training with children. *Journal of Psychology and Psychiatry, 26,* 17-41.

Peplau, H. (1994). Quality of life: An interpersonal perspective. *Nursing Science Quarterly, 7*(1), 10-15.

Pike, A.W. (1991). Moral outrage and moral discourse in nurse-physician collaboration. *Journal of Professional Nursing, 7*(6), 351-362.

Plocher, D.W. (1996). Disease management. In P.R. Kongstvedt (Ed.), *The managed health care services* (3rd ed.). Gaithersburg, MD: Aspen Publishers.

Prouty, M.P. (1983). In A.B. Hamric & J. Spross (Eds.), *The clinical nurse specialist in theory and practice*. New York: Grune & Stratton.

Radwin, L.E. (1996). 'Knowing the patient': A review of research on an emerging concept. *Journal of Advanced Nursing, 23*, 1142-1146.

Raudonis, B.M., & Acton, G.J. (1997). Theory-based nursing practice. *Journal of Advanced Nursing, 26*, 138-145.

Redekopp, M.A. (1997). Clinical nurse specialist role confusion: The need for identity. *Clinical Nurse Specialist, 11*(2), 87-91.

Reigle, J. (1996). Ethical decision-making skills. In A.B. Hamric, J.A. Spross, & C.M. Hanson (Eds.), *Advanced nursing practice: An integrative approach* (pp. 273-295). Philadelphia: W.B. Saunders.

Rest, J.R. (1986). Moral development: Advances in research and theory. New York: Praeger.

Roberts, S.J., Tabloski, P., & Bova, C. (1997). Epigenesis of the nurse practitioner role revisited. *Journal of Nursing Education, 36*(2), 67-73.

Rolfe, G. (1997a). Beyond expertise: Theory, practice, and the reflexive practitioner. *Journal of Clinical Nursing, 6*, 93-97.

Rowdin, M.A. (1995). Conflicts in managed care. *New England Journal of Medicine, 332*(9), 604.

Safriet, B.J. (1992). Health care dollars and regulatory sense: The role of advanced practice nursing. *Yale Journal of Regulation, 9*(2), 149-220, 417-487.

Safriet, B.J. (1994). Impediments to progress in health care workforce policy: License and practice laws. *Inquiry, 31*(3), 310-317.

Safriet, B.J. (1998). Still spending dollars, still searching for sense: Advanced practice nursing in an era of regulatory and economic turmoil. *Advanced Practice Nursing Quarterly, 4*(3), 24-33.

Saulo, M., & Wagener, R.J. (1996). How good case managers make tough choices: Ethics and mediation. *Journal of Care Management, 2*(1), 8.

Schön, D.A. (1984). The reflective practitioner: How professionals think in action (2nd ed.). San Francisco: Jossey-Bass.

Schumacher, K., & Meleis, A. (1994). Transitions: A central concept in nursing. *Image: The Journal of Nursing Scholarship, 26*, 119-127.

Schumacher, K.L., & Meleis, A.I. (1994). Transitions: A central concept in nursing. *Image: The Journal of Nursing Scholarship, 26*(2), 119-127.

Shannon, S.E. (1997). The roots of interdisciplinary conflict around ethical issues. *Critical Care Nursing Clinics of North America, 9*(1), 13.

Simpson, R.L. (1998). Bridging the nursing-physician gap: Technology's role in interdisciplinary practice. *Nursing Administration Quarterly, 22*(3), 87-90.

Smeltzer, C.H. (1991). The art of negotiation: An everyday experience. *Journal of Nursing Administration, 21*(7/8), 26-30.

Solomon, M.Z., O'Donnell, L., Jennings, B., Guilfoy, V., Wolf, S.M., Nolan, K., Jackson, R., Koch-Weser, D., & Donnelly, S. (1993). Decisions near the end of life: Professional views on life-sustaining treatments. *American Journal of Public Health, 83*(1), 14-23.

Sparacino, P.S.A. & Cooper, D.M. (1990). The role components. In P.S.A. Sparacino, D.M. Cooper, & P.A. Minarik (Eds.), *The clinical nurse specialist: Implementation and impact* (pp. 11-40). Norwalk, CT: Appleton & Lange.

Spencer, E.M. (1997). A new role for institutional ethics committees: Organizational ethics. *Journal of Clinical Ethics, 8*(4), 372-376.

Spielman, B.J. (1993). Conflict in medical ethics cases: Seeking patterns of resolution. *Journal of Clinical Ethics, 8*(4), 372-376.

Spross, J. (1994). Coaching: An interdisciplinary perspective. Unpublished manuscript, Doctoral Program in Nursing, Boston College.

Spross, J.A. (1989). The CNS as collaborator. In A.B. Hamric & J.A. Spross (Eds.), *The clinical nurse specialist in theory and practice* (2nd ed., pp. 205-226). Philadelphia: W.B. Saunders.

Spross, J.A., & Baggerly, J. (1989). Models of advanced practice. In A.B. Hamric & J.A. Spross (Eds.), *The clinical nurse specialist in theory and practice* (2nd ed., pp. 19-40). Philadelphia: W.B. Saunders.

Spross, J.A., Clarke, E.B., & Beauregard, J. (2000). Expert coaching and guidance. In A.B. Hamric, J.A. Spross, & C.M. Hanson (Eds.), *Advanced nursing practice: An integrative approach* (2nd ed., pp. 183-216). Philadelphia: W. B. Saunders.

Spross, J.A., & Heaney, C.A. (2000). Shaping advanced nursing practice in the new millennium. *Seminars in Oncology Nursing, 16*, 12-24.

Steele, J.E. (Ed.) (1986). *Issues in collaborative practice.* Orlando, FL: Grune & Stratton.

Steele, S., & Fenton, M.V. (1988). Expert practice of clinical nurse specialists. *Clinical Nurse Specialist, 2*, 45-52.

Stetler, C.B. (1985). Research utilization: Defining the concept. *IMAGE: The Journal of Nursing Scholarship, 17*(2), 40-44.

Stetler, C.B., Bautista, C., Vernale-Hannon, C., & Foster, J. (1995). Enhancing research utilization by clinical nurse specialists. *Nursing Clinics of North America, 30,* 457-473.

Stetler, C.B., & DiMaggio, G. (1991). Research utilization among clinical nurse specialists. *Clinical Nurse Specialist, 5*(3), 151-155.

Stetler, C., Morsi, D., Rucki, S., Broughton, S., Corrigan, B., Fitzgerald, J., Giuliano, K., Havener, P., & Sheridan, E.A. (1998). Utilization-focused integrative reviews in a nursing service. *Applied Nursing Research, 11*(4), 195-206.

Styles, M.M. (1998). An international perspective: APN credentialing. *Advanced Practice Nursing Quarterly, 4*(3), 1-5.

Sullivan, T.J. (1998). *Collaboration: A health care imperative.* New York: McGraw-Hill Health Professions Division.

Torres, S., & Dominguez, L.M. (1998). Collaborative practice: How we get from coordination to the integration of skills and knowledge. In C.M. Sheehy & M.C. McCarthy (Eds.), *Advanced practice nursing: Emphasizing common roles* (pp. 217-240). Philadelphia: F.A. Davis.

Toulmin, S. (1994). Casuistry and clinical ethics. In E.R. DuBose, R. Hamel, & L.J. O'Connell (Eds.), *A matter of principles?* (pp. 310-318). Valley Forge, PA: Trinity Press International.

Turner, L.N., Marquis, K., & Burman, M.E. (1996). Rural nurse practitioners: Perceptions of ethical dilemmas. *Journal of the American Academy of Nurse Practitioners, 8*(6), 269.

Urban, N. (1997). Managed care challenges and opportunities for cardiovascular advanced practice nurses. *AACN Clinical Issues, 8,* 78-89.

Ury, W. (1993). *Getting past no.* New York: Bantam Books.

van Hooft, S. (1990). Moral education for nursing decisions. *Journal of Advanced Nursing, 15,* 210.

Waite, M.S., Harker, J.O., & Messerman, L.I. (1994). Interdisciplinary team training and diversity: Problems, concepts and strategies. In D. Wieland et al (Eds.), *Cultural diversity and geriatric health care: Challenges to the health care professions* (pp. 65-82). New York: Haworth Press.

Ward, M.D., & Rieve, J.A. (1997). The role of care management in disease management. In W.E. Todd & D. Nash (Eds.), *Disease management: A systems approach to improving patient outcomes* (pp. 235-259). Chicago: American Hospital Publishing.

Warden, G.L. (1997). Future organizational leadership. *Journal of Professional Nursing, 13*(6), 334.

Watson, J. (1997). The theory of human caring: Retrospective and prospective. *Nursing Science Quarterly, 10,* 49-52.

Weiss, M. (1998). Case management as a tool for clinical integration. *Advanced Practice Nursing Quarterly, 4*(1), 9-15.

Weiss, M.E. (1998). Case management as a tool for clinical integration. *Advanced Practice Nursing Quarterly, 4*(1), 9-15.

Williams, J.K., & Lea, D.H. (1995). Applying new genetic technologies: Assessment and ethical considerations. *Nurse Practitioner, 20*(7), 16, 21-26.

Williamson, S.H. & Hutcherson, C. (1998). Mutual recognition: Response to the regulatory implications of a changing health care environment. *Advanced Practice Nursing Quarterly, 4*(3), 86-93.

Winters, G., Glass, E., & Sakurai, C. (1993). Ethical issues in oncology nursing practice: An overview of topics and strategies. *Oncology Nursing Forum, 20*(Suppl. 10), 21-34.

York, R., Brown, L.P., Samuels, P., Finkler, S.A., Jacobsen, B., Perseley, C.A., Swank, A., & Robbins, D. (1997). A randomized trial of early discharge and nurse specialist transitional follow-up care of high-risk childbearing women. *Nursing Research, 46*(5), 254-261.

Zaner, R.M. (1988). *Ethics and the clinical encounter.* Englewood Cliffs, NJ: Prentice-Hall.

CNS Certification Questions

1. The ANA social policy statement defines the components of CNS expansion as
    a. new practice skills and knowledge.*
    b. graduation from a Master's program.
    c. care of patients and families as a major focus.
    d. use of research as basis for practice.

2. The ANA would classify the following as advanced practice nurses
    a. Head Nurse and Quality Assurance Nurse.
    b. CNS and NP.*
    c. CNS and Head Nurse.
    d. NP and Quality Improvement Nurse.

3. The central activities of the APN are diagnosis and treatment of complex responses to actual or potential health problems, prevention of illness and injury, provision of comfort, and
    a. rehabilitation.
    b. interpreting X-rays.
    c. maintenance of health.*
    d. facilitating death.

4. The three primary criteria for advanced practice as a CNS are a graduate degree in advanced nursing practice, focus on patient/family, and
    a. consultation abilities.
    b. administrative competency.
    c. interpersonal skills.
    d. professional certification.*

5. All advanced practice nurses share common competencies that include consultation, research skills, expert guidance and coaching of patients/families, collaboration, clinical and professional leadership, and which of the following?
    a. family counseling.
    b. physical assessment.
    c. ethical decision making.*
    d. group therapy.

6. What authority defines the scope of practice of the CNS?
    a. legal.*
    b. political.
    c. religious.
    d. educational.

7. Who defines the scope of practice of the CNS when he/she moves from one state to another?
   a. each state he/she lives in.*
   b. by agreements between states in a region.
   c. a national standard.
   d. an international agreement.

8. The four dimensions of CNS practice are clinical expert, educator, researcher, and which of the following?
   a. direct care provider.
   b. consultant.*
   c. family liaison.
   d. counselor.

9. The unique feature of the blended CNS/NP is his/her ability to provide
   a. primary care.
   b. hospital based care.
   c. outpatient care.
   d. care across settings.*

10. The focus of practice of the blended CNS/NP is patients/families, organizations, and
    a. nursing staff.*
    b. medical staff.
    c. administration.
    d. ancillary nursing staff.

11. The CNS differs from the specialist in that the specialist
    a. focuses on a delineated population or disease.
    b. provides for diagnosis and treatment.
    c. involves patient as well as family.
    d. lacks graduate preparation as an APN.*

12. APNs are differentiated from basic nurses by which of the following?
    a. specialization.
    b. expansion.
    c. advancement.
    d. all of the above.*

13. The specialty group for CNSs is
    a. Joint Commission on Accreditation of Healthcare Organizations (JCAHO).
    b. National League for Nurses (NLN).
    c. National Association of Clinical Nurse Specialists (NACNS).*
    d. American Nurses Association (ANA).

14. In the novice-to-expert model, regression to a lower stage of performance is anticipated under what circumstances?
    a. the CNS enters a familiar situation.
    b. the CNS functions without intense supervision.
    c. the CNS enters a new position.*
    d. the CNS supervises a CNS student.

15. In the Dreyfus novice-to-expert model of skill acquisition, the CNS that is able to appraise a clinical situation holistically is best described as:
    a. a novice.
    b. competent.
    c. proficient.*
    d. an expert.

16. In role development, blurring of responsibilities, uncertainty about implementation of the various aspects of the role, and lack of clarity of expectations are characteristics of role:
    a. conflict.
    b. incongruity.
    c. ambiguity.*
    d. distress.

17. Intraprofessional role conflict exists between the CNS and
    a. nursing staff.*
    b. PT, OT, Nutritionist.
    c. Administrators.
    d. Physicians.

18. Transition into the CNS role is facilitated when the CNS has a choice whether to move into the role, sufficient time and energy to do anticipatory planning support for the change, and has
    a. many years of experience as an RN.
    b. a family member who has had a similar role.
    c. knowledge and skills appropriate to the job.*
    d. no expectations of the role.

19. Rehearsal of situations that the CNS expects to encounter in practice can result in decreased role
    a. ambiguity.
    b. incongruity.
    c. strain.*
    d. conflict.

20. Role playing, psychodrama, case studies, and making rounds on the population of interest assists the CNS student in
    a. values clarification.
    b. role acquisition.*
    c. role definition.
    d. life transitions.

21. Direct patient care activities are the central component of the CNS role. These activities include teaching-coaching, helping patients and families during crisis, and
    a. critically analyzing relevant literature.
    b. writing policies and procedures.
    c. monitoring therapeutic interventions.*
    d. participating in committee meetings.

22. The partnership of the CNS and patient are determined by the duration of the relationship, the cultural background of each, and
    a. institutional policy.
    b. patient preference.*
    c. potential patient outcomes.
    d. the educational level of the patient.

23. The CNS is unable to enter fully into a partnership with patients who are very young, have compromised cognitive capacity, or are
    a. unconscious.*
    b. outpatient.
    c. home care patients .
    d. difficult to manage.

24. Based on the intuitive school, expert clinical skill and performance are best characterized as
    a. an assessment-diagnosis-treatment model.
    b. perceiving-sensing-understanding perspectives.*
    c. information-processing viewpoints.
    d. domain specific.

25. The initial activity utilized by the CNS in expert clinical thinking is
    a. hypothesis formation.
    b. scanning the situation.*
    c. developing a plan.
    d. performing focused assessment.

26. Treatment decisions made by the CNS are complex. All of the following probability characteristics are optimal *except*
    a. high cost.*
    b. treatment effectiveness.
    c. low risk.
    d. patient-specific effectiveness.

27. The key to individualized patient care is knowing
    a. facility resources.
    b. the research literature.
    c. the patient.*
    d. family preferences.

28. Preventive ethics consists of decision-making, ethical considerations, and critical thinking. This approach emphasizes
    a. subjective analysis.
    b. retrospective case analysis.
    c. averting conflict prior to its development.*
    d. shadowing the healthcare provider to understand his/her actions.

29. Synthesis of scientific knowledge can be found in various clinical journals as integrative research reviews, meta-analyses, and
    a. case study analysis.
    b. research-based clinical guidelines.*
    c. seminal research.
    d. clinical exemplars.

30. Middle range theories are more applicable than conceptual models for the CNS because middle range theories
    a. are more abstract.
    b. provide a bigger picture of the issue.
    c. are more specific.*
    d. are prescriptive.

31. Often multiple medical teams manage a patient cared for by a CNS, resulting in conflicting goals and interventions. A CNS facilitates positive patient outcomes when he/she
    a. provides patient comfort.
    b. facilitates communication.*
    c. takes over a patient's care management.
    d. notifies administration there is a problem.

32. Developmental transitions that reflect life cycle transitions include all except
    a. adolescence.
    b. aging.
    c. parenting.
    d. pregnancy.*

33. Successful transitions facilitated by the CNS are characterized by
    a. subjective well being.
    b. well-being of relationships.
    c. role mastery.
    d. all of the above.*

34. The relationship between patient and CNS during coaching is best characterized as
    a. distant.
    b. therapeutic.*
    c. emotionally involved.
    d. objective.

35. Successful coaching by the CNS to facilitate the patient/client's adaptation to their new condition, situation, disease related role is best described as
    a. passive.
    b. dependent.
    c. involved.*
    d. aggressive.

36. In planning what coaching strategy to use to enhance the patient's cognitive knowledge of a newly diagnosed chronic illness, the CNS should consider that what percentage of adults have reading and math limitations which affect their ability to perform activities of daily living?
    a. 75%.
    b. 50%.*
    c. 25%.
    d. 10%.

37. Consultation is defined as
    a. where the clinician relinquishes responsibility for the patient's plan of care.
    b. expert opinion without authority for management.*
    c. one professional manages some aspect of care, while another professional does not.
    d. an ongoing supportive and educational process between a senior and expert clinician and less senior clinician.

38. Supervision is defined as
    a. where the clinician relinquishes responsibility for the patient's plan of care.
    b. expert opinion without authority for management.
    c. one professional manages some aspect of care, while another professional does not.
    d. ongoing supportive and educational process between a senior and expert clinician and less senior clinician.*

39. Co-Management is defined as
    a. the clinician relinquishing responsibility for the patient's plan of care.
    b. expert opinion without authority for management.
    c. one professional managing some aspect of care, while another professional does not.*
    d. an ongoing supportive and educational process between a senior and expert clinician and less senior clinician.

40. The CNS is called as a consultant to evaluate an education approach to a large chronically ill population. The focus of this evaluation is the substantive content and how it is presented. You would call this CNS a
    a. consultee centered consultant.
    b. patient/client centered.
    c. administrative centered consultant.
    d. program centered consultant.*

41. An important legal consideration for CNS consultant documentation includes:
    a. clinical accountability.
    b. accountability for recommendations.*
    c. fiscal accountability.
    d. consultee accountability.

42. Most consultation undertaken by the CNS is provided to
    a. staff nurses.*
    b. physicians.
    c. families.
    d. interdisciplinary team members.

43. Research utilization involves
    a. developing research protocols.
    b. analyzing data.
    c. critiquing and incorporating research.*
    d. consenting subjects for a study.

44. In conducting research, the CNS has many functions that may include
    a. incorporating relevant research into practice.
    b. recruitment of subjects.*
    c. publishing study findings.
    d. evidence-based practice.

45. The competency fundamental to all levels of research activity of the CNS is:
    a. review and critical analysis of the literature.*
    b. participating in research.
    c. identifying nurse-sensitive outcomes.
    d. developing a research protocol.

46. Transactional leadership is:
    a. when one person fosters the exchange of something of value.*
    b. when leadership is situationally based and roles change based on environmental demands.
    c. a participating process that legitimizes situational leadership.
    d. where the purposes of the leader and follower become fused, creating unity of purpose.

47. Transformational leadership is:
    a. when one person fosters the exchange of something of value.
    b. when leadership is situationally based and roles change based on environmental demands.
    c. a participating process that legitimizes situational leadership.
    d. where the purposes of the leader and follower become fused, creating unity of purpose.*

48. The CNS leader who goes outside the usual employment system to create new opportunities for their special expertise is utilizing what type of leadership?
    a. Clinical.
    b. entrepreneurial.*
    c. organizational.
    d. all of the above.

49. Classic models of change, e.g., Lewin, Big Three Model, Bridges, have limited value today because they:
    a. are complex.
    b. require planned change.
    c. are linear.*
    d. are outdated.

50. The CNS undertakes a change project related to a procedure that is often performed in his/her population. The CNS can identify successful leadership in the situation where a project fails by which of the following?
    a. submission of his/her resignation.
    b. reassessment and revision of the project.*
    c. withdrawing further participation in the project.
    d. taking omnipotent control.

51. The essential measure of a successful CNS mentor is:
    a. helping others to grow.*
    b. an award from management.
    c. financial gain.
    d. promotion.

52. Key to successful CNS leadership is
    a. overcoming conflict.*
    b. being "liked" by the staff.
    c. completing tasks independently.
    d. supporting competition among the staff.

53. The hallmark of good collaboration is:
    a. never disagreeing.
    b. always being pleasant.
    c. shared professional interaction.*
    d. a strong social relationship.

54. The most important result of good collaboration is:
    a. improved job satisfaction.
    b. definition of CNS territory.
    c. positive patient outcomes.*
    d. efficient patient care.

55. The most important reason that physicians and CNS' collaborate is that it:
    a. reduces competition.
    b. costs less.
    c. is an ethical imperative.*
    d. provides divergent perspectives.

56. Within clinical practice, an ethical moral dilemma is present when in a given clinical situation, there:
    a. are two acceptable alternatives.*
    b. is one clearly correct answer to the issue.
    c. is a significant need for external consultation.
    a. the CNS lacks authority for the solution.

57. Knowledge development, the first phase in the core competencies for ethical-moral decision making, requires which of the following as central to this phase?
    a. ethical theories and issues common to the population.*
    b. mentoring/facilitating strategies.
    c. role modeling.
    d. working with the team to make decisions.

58. Responding to ethical issues, the CNS pursues:
    a. moral action.*
    b. legal action.
    c. informal resolution.
    d. formal communication.

59. Which of the following phrases best captures the principle of nonmaleficence?
    a. respect for personal values.
    b. do no harm.*
    c. tell the truth.
    d. do good.

60. Which of the following phrases best captures the principle of beneficence?
    a. respect for personal values.
    b. do no harm.
    c. tell the truth.
    d. do good.*

61. Which of the following phrases best captures the principle of autonomy?
    a. respect for personal values.*
    b. do no harm.
    c. tell the truth.
    d. do good.

62. Judgment in the casuistic model of ethical decision-making is based on which of the following?
    a. principles.
    b. rules.
    c. paradigm cases.*
    d. law.

63. The casuistic model is best described as which of the following?
    a. inductive.*
    b. deductive.
    c. not related to a specific context.
    d. virtue base theory.

64. Successful resolution of moral issues cannot occur without:
    a. knowledge of the context of the issue.
    b. knowledge of the right course of action.
    c. moral action by those involved.*
    d. persistence.

65. Issues that involve some form of controversy about moral values are by definition
    a. administrative concerns.
    b. communication problems.
    c. related to insufficient knowledge.
    d. ethical dilemmas.*

66. The CNS who acts as a mediator
    a. suggests various solutions to resolve the issue.
    b. identifies acceptable plans.
    c. offers his/her opinion of what is right.
    d. guides without taking a position.*

67. When collaboration is used to achieve moral resolution, emotions are best
    a. suppressed.
    b. verbalized.*
    c. acted out.
    d. criticized.

68. Compromise as an approach to moral resolution is used when all the following are true *except*
    a. both parties possess a high level of moral certainty in their position.
    b. there is no desire to preserve the relationship.*
    c. time for resolution is limited.
    d. both parties are willing to waive some components under consideration.

69. Accommodation is used to resolve moral conflict when:
    a. there is no commitment to the ongoing relationship.
    b. time is not limited.
    c. the issue is considered significant.*
    d. both parties have a high level of moral certainty.

70. When coercion is used to resolve an issue, it results in
    a. valuing the other person's perspective.
    b. damage to the self-esteem of the person controlled.*
    c. passiveness on the part of the person who is controlled.
    d. equal sharing of decision making power.

71. Evaluation of the outcomes of ethical decision-making focuses on examination of:
    a. problems encountered in the dispute.
    b. interaction between the involved parties.
    c. consequences of the action(s) taken.*
    d. the issue in dispute.

72. The direct care role of the CNS provides him/her the opportunity to:
    a. establish standards of care.
    b. developing a critical pathway.
    c. care for a problematic patient.*
    d. substitute for the staff nurse for breaks.

73. Indirect care provided by the CNS may include:
    a. championing a clinical pathway.
    b. collaboration with the health team to develop standards of care.
    c. examination of recurrent patient problems.
    d. all of the above.*

74. An example of internal consultation is:
    a. identifying barriers to implementation of a facility wide disaster plan.*
    b. writing an article for publication on a frequently encountered disease.
    c. being president of a specialty organization.
    d. sitting on the board of a volunteer health organization.

75. Evidence based practice requires the CNS to:
    a. evaluate the literature relevant to his/her population.*
    b. identify researchable problems.
    c. participate in on-going research.
    d. manipulate the internal validity of the research.

76. The sphere of influence unique to the CNS when compared with that of the NP or midwife is:
    a. care of the patient/client and his/her family.
    b. facilitating the work of the organization/network.*
    c. commitment to a professional organization.
    d. influence on patient/client centered outcomes.

77. Outcome data are used by the CNS for analyzing which of the following?
    a. interdisciplinary communication.
    b. system functions.
    c. coordination of care.
    d. all of the above.*

78. While the debate between staff and line position continues, it is important to remember that the advantage of the CNS in a line position is that it
    a. has fewer administrative responsibilities.
    b. focuses more on patient care.
    c. has formal authority.*
    d. uses only part of available clinical time.

79. Multi-site licensure provides the authority for which of the following?
    a. The nurse licensed to practice in one state to practice in participating states.*
    b. The nurse licensed to practice in one state to practice anywhere in the United States.
    c. The CNS licensed to practice in one state to practice in participating states.
    d. The CNS licensed to practice in one state to practice anywhere in the United States.

80. The Advanced Practice Nurse Case Manager (APNCM) differs from the traditional CNS in that the APNCM is responsible for:
    a. care of individuals.
    b. education of patients/families.
    c. care strategies across the continuum of care.*
    d. setting goals mutually acceptable to the patient and the health team.

81. Regulatory constraints of a cost-managed system include all of the following *except*
    a. utilization review.
    b. realization of profit margins for stockholders.*
    c. a quality improvement program.
    a. selection standards for care providers.

82. To achieve the greatest reduction in costs, the APNCM must target which population of chronically ill patients?
    a. those with no active symptoms.
    b. those who are stable and require episodic care.
    c. those who do not practice behaviors to limit disease and prevent complications.*
    d. those with terminal illness.

83. The APNCM's goal in disease management for those with chronic illness is:
    a. control costs, limit complications.*
    b. cure the disease, limit complications.
    c. control costs, cure the disease.
    d. control costs, cure the disease, limit complications.

84. Measurement of changes in utilization patterns as an outcome of care in chronic illness is best measured with
    a. serial blood work on relevant parameters.
    b. patient satisfaction.
    c. readmission rate.*
    d. cost.

85. You would describe the certification and individual scope of practice regulations from one advanced nursing role to another as:
    a. uniform within each state.
    b. uniform across the United States.
    c. uniform within each state but variable between states.
    d. inconsistent within and between states.*

86. The scope of practice for the CNS refers to
    a. what the CNS can do to/for patients.
    b. what the CNS can delegate.
    c. when collaboration is required.
    d. all of the above.*

87. Who sets standards of practice for CNSs?
    a. professional organizations.*
    b. hospital or facility of employment .
    c. the state board that regulates nursing practice.
    d. research as seen in evidence based practice.

88. State licensure for the APN is designed primarily to:
    a. increase state income.
    b. guarantee the safety of the public.*
    c. protect the nurse.
    d. prevent law suits.

89. Prescriptive authority for the APN is granted by
    a. facilities, clinics, or hospitals where the APN practices.
    b. state board of nurse registration.
    c. interstate agreements.
    d. national certification.

90. National certification as a requirement to practice as an APN is
    a. required in all states.
    b. required for international practice.
    c. required in some states.*
    d. required by inter-state agreements.

91. After initial national APN certification is obtained through testing, recertifications is:
    a. not required as certification is for life.
    b. required annually.
    c. required at regular intervals.*
    d. based on state requirements for continuing education credits.

92. Collaborative practice arrangements between physicians and APNs formalized in a written agreement protect:
    a. the physician.
    b. the APN.
    c. the patient.
    d. all of the above.*

93. Standards for institutional credentialing of an APN are set by:
    a. the facility's joint practice committee.*
    b. the facility's chief operating officer.
    c. the city health code in which practice takes place.
    d. the state board of nurse registration.

CNS Certification Answers

1. a. Correct: Expansion refers to acquiring new knowledge and skills that legitimize role autonomy.
   b. Incorrect: Graduation for a Masters program with a focus in clinical nursing is part of advanced practice but does not define expansion.
   c. Incorrect: Care of patients and families is the focus of advanced practice but does not define expansion.
   d. Incorrect: Use of research as the basis for practice is part of advanced practice but does no define expansion.

2. a. Incorrect: Neither role is advanced clinical practice.
   b. Correct: Both the CNS and NP are advanced practice nurses.
   c. Incorrect: The level of clinical practice of a CNS is advanced but the head nurse is not necessarily an advanced practice nurse.
   d. Incorrect: The NP is an advanced practice nurse. The Quality Improvement nurse may not necessarily provide direct patient care at the advanced practice level.

3. a. Incorrect: Rehabilitation is part of treatment of actual health problems.
   b. Incorrect Interpreting x-rays is part of diagnosis of actual or potential health problems.
   c. Correct: This is the definition provided in ANA's Scope and Standards of Advanced Practice Registered Nursing (1996).
   d. Incorrect: Providing comfort is an important role but not facilitating death.

4. a. Incorrect. Consultation is an advanced practice skill, not one of the primary criteria.
   b. Incorrect. Administrative skills are important, but not one of the primary criteria.
   c. Incorrect. Interpersonal skills are important for the CNS but they are not one of the primary criteria.
   d. Correct: Professional certification tells the consumer that the CNS is competent for advanced practice nursing. Not all areas of practice have advanced practice certification examinations but increasingly they are being developed.

5. a. Incorrect. Family counseling done by the CNS is considered part of expert guidance and coaching.
   b. Incorrect: Physical assessment is a central ingredient of direct clinical practice.
   c. Correct: Fundamental to advanced practice is an ethical perspective that results in ethical decision-making.
   d. Incorrect: Group therapy is part of expert guidance and coaching. In some CNSs' practice, it may be a dominant activity.

6. a. Correct: The Board of Nurse Registration in each state defines the scope of practice for CNSs. In some states, this board is combined with the medical or pharmacy board.
   b. Incorrect: Political authority may influence how the law in each state is formulated but it has only informal influence on advanced practice.
   c. Incorrect: Religious authority may influence how the law for advanced practice is written e.g., participation in abortions, fetal surgery, end of life issues. Religious leaders however, do not have authority for advanced practice.
   d. Incorrect: The National League for Nursing traditionally has accredited graduate nursing programs. There is no educational authority per se. ANP programs have been influenced by internal processes (e.g., W.K. Kellogg Foundation) and internal forces (e.g., American Association of Colleges of Nursing).

7. a. Correct: When a CNS moves or wants to become certified in another state, authority must be sought from each state's board of nurse registration.
   b. Incorrect: Agreements exist between some states and regions but they apply only to the basic registered nurse and not to the advanced practice nurse.
   c. Incorrect: A national standard for CNS certification does not exist, although it has been sought for a number of years.
   d. Incorrect: CNSs who are recognized in another country must seek certification in the state in which he/she wishes to practice.

8. a. Incorrect. Direct and indirect care are dimensions of expert clinical practice.
   b. Correct: Consultation allows the CNS to communicate knowledge on request without having authority over how the person seeking the consultation acts.
   c. Incorrect: Being a family liaison is an important part of clinical expertise. The family liaison role often is required in times of life threatening illness, when there is disagreement among the family about how aggressive care should be pursued.
   d. Incorrect: The counselor role is a dimension of clinical expertise and education as it allows the CNS to help patients/families understand treatment/care options without indicating which to select.

9. a. Incorrect: Primary care is a part of NP education but primary care could be provided by a CNS e.g., diabetes, cardiovascular.
   b. Incorrect: Hospital based care is an integral part of the traditional CNS role.
   c. Incorrect: The CNS or NP can provide setting-specific care. Outpatient care is traditionally the role of the NP but some CNSs are prepared to care for patients in this arena.
   d. Correct: Cross-setting care that incorporates primary care and a focus on the population and care-giving personnel is a characteristic of the blended role.

10. a. Correct: The nursing staff is the focus of education by those in the blended role.
    b. Incorrect: The medical staff is not the primary focus of the advanced practice nurse in the blended role.
    c. Incorrect: Administration is not the primary focus of the advanced practice nurse in the blended role, although they may be a group to whom the advanced practice nurse reports.
    d. Incorrect: Ancillary staff is important but they are not a primary focus of the CNS/NP.

11. a. Incorrect: Both the CNS and specialist focus on a delineated population or disease.
    b. Incorrect: Both provide diagnosis and treatment.
    c. Incorrect: Both are involved with the patient as well as the family.
    d. Correct: The specialist is not masters prepared in a clinical focus. Commonly the specialist is a bachelor's prepared person with rich clinical experience.

12. a. Incorrect: Specialization is one characteristic of the APN but it is only one of the characteristics.
    b. Incorrect: Expansion is one way to differentiate the basic nurse and APN.
    c. Incorrect: Advancement is one characteristic of the APN but is only one of several differences that exist.
    d. Correct: All three of these characteristics differentiate the basic nurse from the APN.

13. a. Incorrect: JCAHO accredits hospitals, home care, and hospice.
    b. Incorrect: The NLN accredits schools of nursing.
    c. Correct: The NACNS is the national specialty group that addresses CNS concerns, regardless of the substantive specialty.
    d. Incorrect: The ANA is the national professional organization for nursing. Its affiliates include many specialty groups e.g., Oncology Nurses Society (ONS), American Association of Critical Care Nurses (AACN).

14. a. Incorrect: Entering a familiar situation allows the CNS to function comfortably at his/her existing performance level.
    b. Incorrect: Independent function of the CNS does not lead to regression to an earlier stage of performance. On the other hand, intense supervision may result in regression to a lower level of performance.
    c. Correct: Entering a new position results in regression to a lower level of function. Factors such as appraising the setting, getting to know the personnel, and evaluating the expectations have been related to this regression. Once the new environment is understood, the CNS can return to his/her higher level of performance.
    d. Incorrect: Supervision of a student provides the opportunity to model CNS practice and verbalize the thinking behind actions. It does not result in regression.

15. a. Incorrect: A novice is theory driven.
    b. Incorrect: Analytic reasoning drives decisions in this phase.
    c. Correct: The proficient CNS is able to take in the entire situation and see it holistically, while at the same time examining its component parts.
    d. Incorrect. Deliberative rationality characterizes the expert.

16. a. Incorrect: Role conflict is where role expectations are perceived to be contradictory or mutually exclusive.
    b. Incorrect: Role incongruity is intrarole conflict. It comes either from lack of skills or knowledge to meet the obligations of the role or from lack of compatibility between personal values and role expectations.
    c. Correct: Role ambiguity results from lack of clarity of the role.
    d. Incorrect: Role distress is when the CNS is unhappy in the role, regardless of the etiology of the distress.

17. a. Correct: Nursing staff and a CNS may experience conflict because there is staff resistance to change, complacency/apathy, or because nurses are not accustomed to seeking consultation from a CNS.
    b. Incorrect: Conflict between the CNS and a physical therapist, occupational therapist, or nutritionist is interprofessional conflict.
    c. Incorrect: Conflict between the CNS and administrators is interprofessional conflict.
    d. Incorrect: Conflict between the CNS and physicians is interprofessional conflict.

18. a. Incorrect: Experience is an asset for the CNS but experience does not make a CNS. Increased knowledge and skills due to years of experience produce a specialist.
    b. Incorrect: Much can be learned from others about the role. Having a family member who has the role similar to the CNS does not inherently facilitate a CNS's transition to the role.
    c. Correct: Knowledge and skills appropriate to the job are pivotal to transition into the CNS role.
    d. Incorrect: The CNS who does not have expectations about the nature of the role in a given situation will have a more difficult transition.

19. a. Incorrect: Role ambiguity is lack of clarity about the expectations of the role.
    b. Incorrect. Role incongruity is intrarole conflict.
    c. Correct: Role strain can be manipulated by reviewing the meaning of the transition, planning, identifying needed knowledge and skills, and expectations of the role. The CNS then can rehearse how to use these in the new situation.
    d. Incorrect: Role conflict is when role expectations are contradictory.

20. a. Incorrect. Values clarification is an internal process by which the CNS re-examines his/her own perspective.
    b. Correct: Strategies such as these provide anticipatory socialization, especially while a graduate student.
    c. Incorrect: Role definition is provided, to a large extent, by job description and these strategies will not alter it.\
    d. Incorrect. Life transitions include growing old, death, marriage, and divorce.

21. a. Incorrect: Critically analyzing literature is an indirect patient care activity.
    b. Incorrect: Writing policies and procedures is an indirect patient care activity.
    c. Correct: Monitoring therapeutic interventions is central to the CNS direct care activity.
    d. Incorrect: Participating in committee meetings is an indirect patient care activity.

22. a. Incorrect: Relationships cannot be dictated by institutional policy.
    b. Correct: Patient preference is pivotal to the relationship with the CNS. It is important that the CNS not make any assumptions about how actively the patient wants to participate in decision-making.
    c. Incorrect: Relationships are not driven by whether the patient will live or die or have complications.
    d. Incorrect: The CNS must be able to communicate and form a therapeutic relationship with persons of all levels of education.

23. a. Correct: When patients are unable to enter into a relationship because of their functional ability, the CNS must pay attention to their cues as to their preference and talk with families/surrogates.
    b. Incorrect: Being an outpatient does not preclude the development of a patient-CNS relationship.
    c. Incorrect: Being a home care patient does not preclude the development of a patient-CNS relationship.
    d. Incorrect: Being a patient that is difficult to manage does not preclude the development of a patient-CNS relationship.

24. a. Incorrect: The assessment-diagnosis-treatment model is the paradigm for critical thinking in the information processing school.
    b. Correct: The innovative school's paradigm for critical thinking follows the perceiving-sensing-understanding approach.
    c. Incorrect: An information-processing viewpoint uses the assessment-diagnosis-treatment model.
    d. Incorrect: Critical thinking in the intuitive school is not domain specific.

25. a. Incorrect: Hypothesis formation can only occur after data are gathered and organized.
    b. Correct: The starting point in critical thinking is obtaining an overview of the situation through record review, physical examination, and the patient's expressed and unexpressed concerns.
    c. Incorrect: Planning occurs after data gathering, hypothesis formation and focused assessment.
    d. Incorrect: Focused assessment allows for confirmation or refuting of hypotheses so diagnosis and planning can take place.

26. a. Correct: High patient costs are not a goal of treatment decisions.
    b. Incorrect: The treatment selected is known to be effective.
    c. Incorrect: Ideally the treatment selected has low or an acceptable risk of complications.
    d. Incorrect: Knowing what has been effective for a patient in the past often is an aid to selection of current treatment.

27. a. Incorrect: Facility resources do not limit the plan or care. If additional/different equipment or supplies are needed, they can be accessed.
    b. Incorrect: Knowing what the literature recommends provides the CNS knowledge of the array of treatment options. It does not reveal what is correct for a specific patient.
    c. Correct: The key to individual patient care is knowing the patient and his/her goals and preferences for care.
    d. Incorrect: While family preferences are important, patient goals and preferences are decisive in individualized care.

28. a. Incorrect: Objectivity about an ethical conflict is part of the role of the CNS.
    b. Incorrect: Retrospective care analysis is informative but will not prevent anything.
    c. Correct: The key to preventive ethics is addressing the situation before it develops into a conflict. For example, it important to clarify an order for a "Full Code" in a vegetative patient before his/her cardiac arrest.
    d. Incorrect: Shadowing the provider will elicit information about critical thinking but is not a requirement of actualizing preventive ethics.

29. a. Incorrect: Case study analyses are limited in their scope, review, and scientific analysis.
    b. Correct: Research-based clinical guidelines are based on expert consensus, strength of scientific evidence, and logical reasoning.
    c. Incorrect: Seminal research is pioneering but requires further exploration.
    d. Incorrect: A clinical exemplar is primarily a single case study and cannot be considered generalizable.

30. a. Incorrect: Middle range theory addresses a particular patient population.
    b. Incorrect: A conceptual model provides a bigger picture of the issue than middle range theory.
    c. Correct: Middle range theory addresses the experience of a population and so is more specific than a conceptual model.
    d. Incorrect: Theory does not explain how to act. Theory addresses the range of options.

31. a. Incorrect: Providing patient comfort is important but it will not resolve goal conflict.
    b. Correct: A CNS often acts as a broker between the patient/family and members of the medical team in an effort to develop a plan of care on which all can agree.
    c. Incorrect: The CNS must work with a team to set and accomplish goals
    d. Incorrect: In resolution of disparate treatment goals, administrative intervention is sought only as a last resort.

32. a. Incorrect: Adolescence is a developmental transition.
    b. Incorrect: Aging is a developmental transition.
    c. Incorrect: Parenting is a developmental transition.
    d. Correct: Pregnancy is a health-illness transition.

33. a. Incorrect: Subjective well-being is one of several signs of successful transition but there are others.
    b. Incorrect: Developing good relationships is one of the several signs of successful transition.
    c. Incorrect: Role mastery is one of the signs of successful transition.
    d. Correct: The combination of subjective well-being, good relationships, and role mastery characterize successful transition into the role of the CNS.

34. a. Incorrect: Being distant does not aid in developing a caring relationship with a patient.
    b. Correct: A therapeutic relationship is a caring relationship focused on the patient's needs with the CNS in the professional helping role.
    c. Incorrect: Being emotionally involved interferes with the objectivity needed to assist the patient with his/her health care issues.
    d. Incorrect: A relationship requires investment and so cannot be totally objective.

35. a. Incorrect: The CNS is active rather than passive.
    b. Incorrect: The CNS is not dependent. The focus is on the patients' goals.
    c. Correct: Coaching requires active involvement by the CNS.
    d. Incorrect: The CNS should be active but not aggressive.

36. a. Incorrect: Not this large a percentage of the population has trouble with math and reading such that it interferes with their lives.
    b. Correct: The National Adult Literacy Survey showed that when reading and arithmetic skills are added together, only half of adult Americans have skills sufficient to support activities of daily living.
    c. Incorrect: About 25% are illiterate.
    d. Incorrect: This is an underestimation of the problem.

37. a. Incorrect: The person requesting the consultation retains authority for the patient.
    b. Correct: The consultant gives an opinion but does not control decisions about care.
    c. Incorrect: Comanagement is where two providers each manage some aspect of care.
    d. Incorrect: Clinical supervision is where a new or less experienced clinician is supported and educated by a senior clinician.

38. a. Incorrect: Supervision is not associated with clinical responsibility for patient care.
    b. Incorrect: Consultation is where one gives expert opinion without authority for the patient's management.
    c. Incorrect: Comanagement is where two providers each manage some aspect of care.
    d. Correct: Clinical supervision is where a new or less experienced clinician is supported and educated by a senior clinician.

39. a. Incorrect: In co-management both providers retain responsibility for the patient.
    b. Incorrect: The consultant gives an opinion but does not control decisions about care.
    c. Correct: By definition this answer is co-management. Co-management often occurs when the patient has multiple comorbidities so two or more practitioners care for the patient, each bringing his/her expertise to the patient's care.
    d. Incorrect: Any ongoing supportive educational process between an expert clinician and a less experienced clinician is called supervision.

40. a. Incorrect: This is not consultation to increase knowledge or skills of the person requesting the consultation.
    b. Incorrect: An individual patient/client is not the focus of consultation.
    c. Incorrect: The focus is not how to conduct the program.
    d. Correct: This consultation focuses on planning and presenting the program.

41. a. Incorrect: The consultee remains clinically responsible for the patient.
    b. Correct: CNS consultants are responsible for their practice, including making reasonable recommendations.
    c. Incorrect: Overall consultant responsibility does not include responsibility for financial expenditures or outcomes.
    d. Incorrect: The consultee remains clinically responsible for the patient. If the primary focus is on consultee education, there is no documentation in a patient's medical record.

42. a. Correct: Most consultation is with the nursing staff.
    b. Incorrect: Working with a physician is important but the main focus of the CNS role is in working with nursing staff and the organization.
    c. Incorrect: The CNS often works with the family but more frequently works the staff nurse.
    d. Incorrect: The interdisciplinary team may require consultation from the CNS but it is less frequent than that requested by the nursing staff.

43. a. Incorrect: Developing research protocols is part of designing a research project.
    b. Incorrect: Analyzing data is part of implementing a research project.
    c. Correct: Research utilization requires analysis and critical review of research for incorporation into practice.
    d. Incorrect: Consent is part of conducting research.

44. a. Incorrect: Incorporating research into practice is research utilization.
    b. Correct: Recruitment of subjects is one aspect of conducting a study.
    c. Incorrect: Publishing study findings is done after the study is completed.
    d. Incorrect: Evidence based practice is where research is the foundation of clinical care.

45. a. Correct: The ability to review and critique the literature relevant to the CNS' population is pivotal to all research skills and fundamental to CNS success.
    b. Incorrect: Not all CNSs participate in research.
    c. Incorrect: Identifying nurse-sensitive outcomes for a population is important but not as pivotal as critiquing the literature.
    d. Incorrect: Not all CNSs develop research protocols.

46. a. Correct: Transactional leadership is where the leader supports the political, economic, or psychological values of followers.
    b. Incorrect: This is situational leadership.
    c. Incorrect: This is roving leadership.
    d. Incorrect: This is transformational leadership.

47. a. Incorrect: This is transactional leadership.
    b. Incorrect: This is situational leadership.
    c. Incorrect: This is roving leadership.
    d. Correct: Transformational leadership results in shared vision and empowers the team to work together to accomplish mutual goals.

48. a. Incorrect: Clinical leadership is where the CNS learns with and from others with whom he/she works.
    b. Correct: Entrepreneurial leadership is where the CNS goes outside the traditional employment to create new opportunities.
    c. Incorrect: Organizational leadership is where leaders are formally elected to positions of power.
    d. Incorrect: Only those in the entrepreneurial leadership role seek to create opportunities to use their expertise and access new sources of income.

49. a. Incorrect: Complexity is inherent in change.
    b. Incorrect: Planned change is not a limitation of the models of change.
    c. Correct: Being linear is a limitation because there is not a mechanism for incorporating change in the situation.
    d. Incorrect: Models of change are timeless as they contain principles that are relevant to change in clinical practice.

50. a. Incorrect: The submission of a resignation is not a sign of leadership.
    b. Correct: Successful leadership is characterized by persistence and re-evaluation of the data when an approach does not work.
    c. Incorrect: Leadership can only be provided when the CNS participates in the project.
    d. Incorrect: Leadership can only be provided when the CNS collaborates with others in the project.

51. a. Correct: The main reward for mentorship is enjoying a protégé's success.
    b. Incorrect: An award for mentorship is nice but not essential.
    c. Incorrect: Mentorship is not entered into for money.
    d. Incorrect: A promotion should not be the intended reward for mentorship.

52. a. Correct: Conflict resolution is key to CNS leadership.
    b. Incorrect: It is nice to be liked but not essential to the effectiveness of leadership.
    c. Incorrect: Leadership requires engagement with others, so completing tasks independently cannot be key to CNS leadership.
    d. Incorrect: Competition among staff undermines a cooperative environment.

53. a. Incorrect: Effective collaboration requires honesty and so may involve disagreement.
    b. Incorrect: Always being pleasant is not realistic.
    c. Correct: Collaboration requires professional interaction to bring knowledge and skills to patient care.
    d. Incorrect: A social relationship is unrelated to professional collaboration.

54. a. Incorrect: Job satisfaction may improve or decline but it is not the most important result of good collaboration.
    b. Incorrect: Territoriality and competitiveness increase when collaboration fails.
    c. Correct: Patient outcomes are the most important product of good collaboration.
    d. Incorrect: Efficient care may or may not result from collaboration.

55. a. Incorrect: MD-CNS collaboration has no direct effect in reducing competition.
    b. Incorrect: MD-CNS collaboration may cost either less or more than care without collaboration.
    c. Correct: Professional collaboration is an ethical imperative.
    d. Incorrect: One cannot predict the physician or CNS perspectives merely on the basis of their collaboration.

56. a. Correct: At least two viable options must be available to create an ethical-moral dilemma.
    b. Incorrect: Where there is a single answer to an issue, it poses no dilemma.
    c. Incorrect: The need for consultation may be present with or without an ethical-moral dilemma.
    d. Incorrect: A CNS's lack of authority does not create an ethical-moral dilemma.

57. a. Correct: Knowledge of ethical theories and issues common to the population are fundamental to phase 1, or the knowledge development phase of the core competencies for ethical decision making.
    b. Incorrect: Mentoring is part of phase 3 of the ethical competencies, creating an ethical environment.
    c. Incorrect: Role modeling is part of phase 3 of the ethical competencies, creating an ethical environment.
    d. Incorrect: Working with others in decision-making is application of moral action.

58. a. Correct: Moral action is pivotal to responding to ethical issues.
    b. Incorrect: Legal action may be used but is not primary.
    c. Incorrect: Informal resolution may be used but is not vital.
    d. Incorrect: Formal communication may be used but is not fundamental..

59. a. Incorrect: The principle of autonomy is respect of personal values.
    b. Correct: Nonmaleficance means to do no harm.
    c. Incorrect: The role of veracity is to tell the truth.
    d. Incorrect: Doing good is the principle of beneficience.

60. a. Incorrect: The principle of autonomy is respect of personal values.
    b. Incorrect: Nonmaleficance means do no harm.
    c. Incorrect: The role of veracity is to tell the truth.
    d. Correct: Doing good is the principle of beneficience.

61. a. Correct: The principle of autonomy is respect of personal values.
    b. Incorrect: Nonmaleficance means do no harm.
    c. Incorrect: The role of veracity is to tell the truth.
    d. Incorrect: Doing good is the principle of beneficence.

62. a. Incorrect: Principles are utilized in the principle-based approach.
    b. Incorrect: Rules are utilized in the principle-based approach.
    c. Correct: Paradigm cases provide a standard against which to evaluate the current case.
    d. Incorrect. Law is utilized in the principle-based approach.

63. a. Correct: An inductive approach works from a specific case to the generalizations, or casuists believe ethical decision making emerges from human moral experiences.
  b. Incorrect: A deductive approach works from generalizations to specific cases.
  c. Incorrect: The casuist model examines dilemmas in a context-specific manner.
  d. Incorrect: Virtue-based theory is an alternative process to the casuist model for moral reflection and argument.

64. a. Incorrect: Knowledge of the context of the issue is important for moral resolution of an issue but it is not sufficient alone.
  b. Incorrect: Knowledge of the right course of action is important for moral resolution but knowledge alone is not sufficient for successful moral resolution.
  c. Correct: Moral action is the essential component for moral resolution of an issue.
  d. Incorrect: Persistence is important but it alone may not lead to successful moral resolution of an issue.

65. a. Incorrect: Administrative concerns may exist but they may or may not be related to moral values.
  b. Incorrect: Communication problems do not necessarily involve some type of moral values.
  c. Incorrect: Insufficient knowledge is not necessarily related to controversy about moral values.
  d. Correct: Controversy about moral values is an ethical dilemma.

66. a. Incorrect: Mediators do not suggest resolutions.
  b. Incorrect: Mediators do not define what an acceptable plan would be.
  c. Incorrect: Mediators are neutral.
  d. Correct: CNS mediators guide without taking a position.

67. a. Incorrect: suppressed emotions display themselves as behavior.
  b. Correct: Verbalization of emotion provides data on which a therapeutic strategy can be developed.
  c. Incorrect: Acting out emotions leaves the door open to inaccurate interpretation of meaning.
  d. Incorrect: Emotions are never criticized but rather accepted as an integral part of an individual.

68. a. Incorrect: Compromise is needed when both parties hold a strong position.
  b. Correct: There is no need to compromise if you don't want to preserve the relationship.
  c. Incorrect: Compromise is needed when there is little time to reach resolution in another manner.
  d. Incorrect: By definition, waiving some components under consideration is compromise.

69. a. Incorrect: Giving in, or accommodation, usually is not done unless an ongoing relationship is desired.
  b. Incorrect: Time pressure does not usually result in accommodation.
  c. Correct: Insignificance of an issue allows one party to give in.
  d. Incorrect: Compromise is usually the route of resolution when both parties have a strong position.

70. a. Incorrect: Coercion is not consistent with respect for the other person.
    b. Correct: Coercion threatens the individual who is coerced and their self-concept.
    c. Incorrect: The response of the person who is coerced cannot be predicted. The range of responses is from aggressive to passive.
    d. Incorrect: Compromise is the term used to describe when both parties share equally in the decision-making,

71. a. Incorrect: Process evaluation is used to examine problems encountered in the dispute.
    b. Incorrect: Process evaluation is used to examine the interpersonal process.
    c. Correct: Outcome evaluation is used to examine the consequences of the decision and action taken.
    d. Incorrect: Process evaluation is used to examine the issue in dispute.

72. a. Incorrect: Establishing standards of care is part of the indirect care role of the CNS.
    b. Incorrect: Developing a critical pathway is part of the indirect care role of the CNS.
    c. Correct: Providing care for a problematic patient is part of the direct care role of the CNS.
    d. Incorrect: Substituting for a staff nurse while the staff nurse is on a break is an indirect care role for the CNS.

73. a. Incorrect: This is one way to provide indirect care but it does not encompass the full extent of indirect care.
    b. Incorrect: This is one way to provide indirect care but it does not encompass the full extent of indirect care.
    c. Incorrect: This is one way to provide indirect care but it does not encompass the full extent of indirect care.
    d. Correct: The indirect care role includes developing pathways, establishing standards and examining common patient problems.

74. a. Correct: Internal consultation focuses on issues within the facility.
    b. Incorrect: Writing an article shares expertise beyond the facility and could be called a type of external consultation.
    c. Incorrect: Being active in a professional organization is an example of external consultation.
    d. Incorrect: Being a member of a board of directors is important but is not internal consultation and is only external if the substantive content is related to the CNS's expertise.

75. a. Correct: Evaluation of the literature is pivotal to use of evidence-based practice.
    b. Incorrect: Identifying researchable problems is part of developing a research project.
    c. Incorrect: Participating in on-going research is not required for evidence-based practice.
    d. Incorrect: The CNS consumer of research cannot manipulate the internal validity of the study, only the researcher can.

76. a. Incorrect: Care of the patient/client and family is common to all advanced practice roles.
    b. Correct: Facilitating the work of the organization is unique to the CNS role.
    c. Incorrect: All advanced practice nurses should have a commitment to a professional organization.
    d. Incorrect: All advanced practice nurses are able to identify patient-centered outcomes.

77. a. Incorrect: Interdisciplinary communication is only one type of outcome evaluated by the CNS.
    b. Incorrect: System outcomes is only one type of outcome data evaluated by the CNS.
    c. Incorrect: Information about coordination of care is only one type of outcome data evaluated by the CNS.
    d. Correct: The CNS uses outcome data to access interdisciplinary communication and collaboration, evaluate system outcomes, and monitor patient progress.

78. a. Incorrect: In a staff position the CNS has fewer administrative responsibilities.
    b. Incorrect: The CNS is a staff position focuses more on patient care than if he/she were in a line position.
    c. Correct: Formal authority is one of the advantages of a line position.
    d. Incorrect: The time spend on administrative responsibilities in a line position may dominate and preclude time for patient care.

79. a. Correct: Multi-state agreements allow a basic professional nurse to move between states participating in the agreement.
    b. Incorrect: There is no national licensure.
    c. Incorrect: There is no multi-state licensure for advanced practice nurses.
    d. Incorrect: There is no national licensure for CNSs.

80. a. Incorrect: The APNCM does not provide direct patient care.
    b. Incorrect: Both provide education.
    c. Correct: The APNCM's job is to make a seamless transition for patients between settings.
    d. Incorrect: Both the APNCM and the CNS must work with the patient and members of the health team to set goals that are mutually acceptable.

81. a. Incorrect: Utilization review is part of a cost-managed system.
    b. Correct: Cost-managed systems are designed to realize profits for shareholders but this is not a regulatory constraint.
    c. Incorrect: Explicit standards for quality improvement are part of a managed system.
    d. Incorrect: Selection standards for care providers are a part of a cost-managed system.

82. a. Incorrect: Those with no symptoms typically are active participants in their treatment.
    b. Incorrect: Episodic care has a small impact on outcomes and overall quality of care.
    c. Correct: It us critical to target high utilization/expenditure patients as they will yield the greatest return from case management strategies.
    d. Incorrect: The terminally ill use finite resources and outcomes reasonably are predictable.

83. a. Correct: The case manager's primary concerns are controlling costs and limiting complications.
    b. Incorrect: In disease management, cure is not a realist goal for the case manager.
    c. Incorrect: In disease management, cure is not a realistic goal for the case manager.
    d. Incorrect: In disease management, cure is not a realistic goal for the case manager.

84. a. Incorrect: Relevant blood work will provide clinical data on a specific patient but not utilization information.
    b. Incorrect: Patient satisfaction will not provide information about utilization, only how pleased people are with what was used.
    c. Correct: Readmission rate is a realistic measure of resource utilization.
    d. Incorrect: Cost alone describes how expensive care is, not which components were used or how often.

85. a. Incorrect: There is no uniformity between advanced practice specialties with a state.
    b. Incorrect There is no national scope of practice.
    c. Incorrect: APN roles (NP, CNS, Midwife, CRNA) vary within and between states.
    d. Correct: Certification and scope of practice vary between advanced practice roles both within and between states.

86. a. Incorrect: The scope of practice includes but is not limited to what the nurse can do to/for patients.
    b. Incorrect: The scope of practice includes but is not limited to what the CNS can delegate.
    c. Incorrect: The scope of practice includes but is not limited to when collaboration is required.
    d. Correct: The scope of practice addresses what the CNS can do to/for patients, what the CNS can delegate, and when collaboration is required.

87. a. Correct: Standards of practice are set by professional organizations.
    b. Incorrect: Institutions do not set standards of practice.
    c. Incorrect: The state board of nursing defines nursing practice in all states but some states do not have titling for CNSs. Standards of practice must adhere to state law.
    d. Incorrect: Standards for practice are broad and general while research that leads to evidence based practice usually is quite specific.

88. a. Incorrect: State licensure for CNS does increase state revenue but that is not its purpose.
    b. Correct: Licensure is designed to protect the public.
    c. Incorrect: State licensure is designed to protect patients rather than nurses.
    d. Incorrect: Licensure does not prevent lawsuits.

89. a. Incorrect: The nurse practice act grants prescriptive authority. It cannot be superceded by these agencies.
    b. Correct: A state's nurse practice act grants prescriptive authority.
    c. Incorrect: Interstate agreements regulate basic nurses, not APNs.
    d. Incorrect: There is not a national authority for prescribing. This authority is retained within each state.

90. a. Incorrect: The requirements for practice are set by each state board and are not uniform throughout the United States.
    b. Incorrect: There is no authority that certifies APNs for international practice.
    c. Correct: some state boards of nurse registration require certification while others do not.
    d. Incorrect: Interstate agreements apply only to basic registered nurses, not to APNs.

91. a. Incorrect: Certification is for a finite number of years.
    b. Incorrect: Annual recertification is not required.
    c. Correct: The certifying body sets the time interval for recertification.
    d. Incorrect: Continuing education credits alone do not determine eligibility for recertification.

92. a. Incorrect: Delineating the practice of the APN decreases physician liability but ANPs and patients also are protected.
    b. Incorrect: The APN is protected because her scope of practice is delimited but MDs and patients also are protected.
    c. Incorrect: The patient is protected because who can do what is outlined but MDs and APNs also are protected.
    d. Correct: This agreement provides protection for all parties i.e., the patient, APN, and the physician.

93. a. Correct: Each institution that employs APNs has some structure for approving activities that the APNs can undertake that are delimited under the law.
    b. Incorrect: The chief operating officer ultimately is responsible for practice in the institution but does not personally set the standards.
    c. Incorrect: The city health code has nothing to do with APN credentialing.
    d. Incorrect: The institution must have its APNs function within the law but it can limit practice or expand it, within those limits.

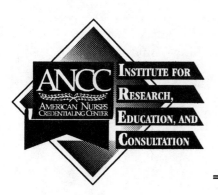

Introduction to Clinical Specialist Addendum

Course CE Application Process

The Institute for Research, Education & Consultation (IREC) of the American Nurses Credentialing Center's (ANCC) announces the *"Clinical Specialist Addendum."* You may earn **6** nursing continuing education contact hours (CH) by completing the application process and following the checklist below. For pricing refer to the current review product catalog or visit our website at www.nursecredentialing.org. Forward payment in full by check or credit card. Make check payable to: ANCC-IREC. The Contact Hour Certificate will be mailed to you within thirty (30) days following receipt of all the information cited in the checklist below and your payment.

INQUIRIES OR COMMENTS

If you have questions about the continuing education contact hours, contact IREC at (202) 651-7252, fax: (202) 488-8190, or by e-mail: bmichels@ana.org. For a duplicate ANCC Nursing Continuing Education Certificate, send a written request with the $5.00 fee. Make checks payable to ANCC-IREC.

To assist you in completing the application process for the IREC's Continuing Education Certificate (for contact hours), use the following checklist:

1. Complete and return the Clinical Nurse Specialist Addendum Registration Form
2. Complete and return the QUESTION ANSWER SHEET
3. Complete and return the Review Course Evaluation Form .
4. Send the completed forms and payment to:

    IREC
    Education Program Specialist
    600 Maryland Avenue SW, Suite 100 West
    Washington, DC 20024-2571

(Note: IREC is accredited as a provider of continuing education in nursing by the Florida Board of Nursing, Provider No. 2943)

Ann Cary, PhD, MPH, RN, A-CCC
Director, IREC

Becky Garcia-Michels, MSN, APRN,BC
Education Program Specialist, IREC

Nursing Continuing Education Reviewers

Marty Cangary
Greenwich, IN

Karen Martin
Los Angeles, CA

Joanne Alderman
Tulsa, OK

The IREC Clinical Specialist Addendum (ME-3) is designed to meet the following objectives:

1. Identify the foundations of the Clinical Nurse Specialist Practice nursing
2. Identify the components of the Clinical Nurse Specialist Practice as expert clinician, educator, consultant, and researcher
3. Explain the key APN Competencies as used by Clinical Nurse Specialists
4. Discuss the CNS in Action as clinical nurse specialist and as the CNS case manager.
5. Describe the Regulatory and Credentialing Requirements for Advanced Practice Nursing

For further information about IREC's Continuing Education and Review Courses call
(202) 651-7252 or visit the website www.nursecredentialing.org

Complete this page if you are requesting Continuing Education Credit.

CERTIFICATION PAGE

Today's Date: _____

Contact Hours: 6

Name: _____

Home Address: _____

City, State, Zip: _____

Home Phone: _____ E-mail: _____

Professional Role Title: _____

Specialty Area of Practice: _____

Institution/Employer: _____

Business Address: _____

City, State, Zip : _____

Business Phone: _____ Fax: _____

Are you a member of your state nurses association? _____ Yes _____ No

Member number: _____

State of RN License and RN License Number: _____

Please list additional state licenses, if applicable: _____

Please list additional certification (s) you currently hold: _____

State in which you are currently practicing: _____

Social Security Number: _____

If you personally purchased this Module please give date (approximate month, year, to help us find your record)._____

If you have not prepaid the Continuing Education fee, please enclose the fee. For pricing please refer to the current review course catalog or visit our website at www.nursecredentialing.org.

Fee enclosed if applicable $_____.

For Credit Card Orders Only: ____VISA ____MASTERCARD _____ EXP. DATE

ACCOUNT NO. _____

Provider approved by the Florida Board of Nursing, Provider No. 2943

Certification of completion will be for 6 Continuing Education Hours. (6 CEH)

Return this page with the Module Evaluation and Quiz Answer Sheet to:

ANCC/IREC

Education Program Specialist

600 Maryland Ave SW, Suite 100 W

Washington, DC 20024-2571

PH: 800-924-9053

CLINICAL NURSE SPECIALIST ADDENDUM **107**

Evaluation Sheet
Clinical Specialist Addendum ME-3

Directions: Please circle the appropriate number which indicates your rating of each statement. Ratings range from 1=low/poor to 5=excellent.

	Low/Poor			High/Excellent		Not Applicable
1. To what extent have you achieved the objectives of this review course?	1	2	3	4	5	N/A
2. To what extent did the content relate to the study objectives?	1	2	3	4	5	N/A
3. To what extent was this teaching method appropriate and aids used effectively?	1	2	3	4	5	N/A

TO WHAT EXTENT DO YOU FEEL THIS INDEPENDENT STUDY MODULE WILL BE:

4. Essential to your area of nursing practice.	1	2	3	4	5	N/A
5. Useful to your area of nursing practice.	1	2	3	4	5	N/A
6. How well does this review course prepare you for the review exam?	1	2	3	4	5	N/A

Which certification exam did you complete?
_____ American Nurses Credentialing Center   _____ Other: _____

Would you be interested in receiving a journal with articles relating to credentialing and continuing education opportunities? _____ Yes _____ No

If yes, which would you prefer? _____ Paper Version _____ Online Version

Which of the following formats would you like to use for future continuing education courses? (Check all that apply)   _____ CD Rom   _____ Web   _____ Audio Cassette

        _____ Compact Disc   _____ Video   _____ On-site course

Total amount of time in minutes it took you to complete the IREC/ANCC "Clinical Specialist Addendum," take and pass the study questions, register and complete the evaluation form:
_____
_____

Comments Welcomed! What other topics would you like to see developed into an independent study module or course for Clinical Nurse Specialists?
_____
_____
_____
_____
_____

Clinical Specialist Addendum
Sample Questions Answer Sheet

Name _____

Today's Date _____

Directions: Circle the correct answer. Comment as needed.

1.	a	b	c	d	32.	a	b	c	d	63.	a	b	c	d
2.	a	b	c	d	33.	a	b	c	d	64.	a	b	c	d
3.	a	b	c	d	34.	a	b	c	d	65.	a	b	c	d
4.	a	b	c	d	35.	a	b	c	d	66.	a	b	c	d
5.	a	b	c	d	36.	a	b	c	d	67.	a	b	c	d
6.	a	b	c	d	37.	a	b	c	d	68.	a	b	c	d
7.	a	b	c	d	38.	a	b	c	d	69.	a	b	c	d
8.	a	b	c	d	39.	a	b	c	d	70.	a	b	c	d
9.	a	b	c	d	40.	a	b	c	d	71.	a	b	c	d
10.	a	b	c	d	41.	a	b	c	d	72.	a	b	c	d
11.	a	b	c	d	42.	a	b	c	d	73.	a	b	c	d
12.	a	b	c	d	43.	a	b	c	d	74.	a	b	c	d
13.	a	b	c	d	44.	a	b	c	d	75.	a	b	c	d
14.	a	b	c	d	45.	a	b	c	d	76.	a	b	c	d
15.	a	b	c	d	46.	a	b	c	d	77.	a	b	c	d
16.	a	b	c	d	47.	a	b	c	d	78.	a	b	c	d
17.	a	b	c	d	48.	a	b	c	d	79.	a	b	c	d
18.	a	b	c	d	49.	a	b	c	d	80.	a	b	c	d
19.	a	b	c	d	50.	a	b	c	d	81.	a	b	c	d
20.	a	b	c	d	51.	a	b	c	d	82.	a	b	c	d
21.	a	b	c	d	52.	a	b	c	d	83.	a	b	c	d
22.	a	b	c	d	53.	a	b	c	d	84.	a	b	c	d
23.	a	b	c	d	54.	a	b	c	d	85.	a	b	c	d
24.	a	b	c	d	55.	a	b	c	d	86.	a	b	c	d
25.	a	b	c	d	56.	a	b	c	d	87.	a	b	c	d
26.	a	b	c	d	57.	a	b	c	d	88.	a	b	c	d
27.	a	b	c	d	58.	a	b	c	d	89.	a	b	c	d
28.	a	b	c	d	59.	a	b	c	d	90.	a	b	c	d
29.	a	b	c	d	60.	a	b	c	d	91.	a	b	c	d
30.	a	b	c	d	61.	a	b	c	d	92.	a	b	c	d
31.	a	b	c	d	62.	a	b	c	d	93.	a	b	c	d